Meditations for Gym Yogis

An Easy Intro to Yoga Philosophy

TERESA BERGEN

ISBN:1494997525
ISBN-13:9781494997526
www.teresabergen.com

Cover art by Anna Magruder

Author photo by Mary Tapogna

This book is dedicated to all my students at West Coast Fitness in Portland, Oregon: those who've come faithfully for years, those who dropped in once, and everybody in between. And especially my Sunday morning classes, who listen to me read.

CONTENTS

ACKNOWLEDGMENTS

I'd like to thank all my teachers and gym and yoga friends, including the many I'm sure to leave out: Jenna Abernathy, Jay Chadney, Terri Chadney, Bill Counter, Tasha Danner, Kimberly Dark, Kathy Elder, Jay Fields, Jenny Gallagher, Jennifer Kapnek, Ginny Kauffman, Monicka Koneski, Molly Long, Simon Menasche, Lisa Mae Osborn, Jennifer Siegel, Jeanie Songer, Tally Thomas, Todd Williamson and Mike Whitehead.

And, always, I appreciate the constant support and encouragement of my parents and sisters.

INTRODUCTION

"The substitute made us Om," complained one of my yoga students when I came back after an absence. Not again, I thought.

I've been teaching at the same gym for more than a decade. Some of my current yoga students predate me and have attended regularly during my whole tenure. Others show up now and then when they need stretching or de-stressing. Many arrive in the yoga room because they're paying for a gym membership and might as well check out all the classes. Some of them stay for years. Others never return.

Their spiritual practices and expectations also vary greatly, at least among those who ever talk to me about their faith. Some are Christian and leery of anything that seems too Hindu. A few are serious Buddhist practitioners who disappear for months at a time to lead or participate in retreats. Not one has ever identified herself as a practicing Hindu. Some are athletes with no apparent interest in spirituality who come to class because they don't stretch enough on their own.

Some students would Om with gusto. Others would head for the door.

I feel most responsible to the newer students, those who are skeptical of yoga, those who don't want to be embarrassed by their inabilities to do poses, those who don't want to suffer through a teacher saying dippy New Age things, or, worse, expecting them to participate in unfamiliar practices they don't understand. I always figure that experienced yoga students who come to my class and find it wanting will go find another teacher. But newbies traumatized by a first yoga experience might never return to any class. In which case, I believe they'll be missing a lot. I certainly don't want to be the one who drove them away from yoga.

While yoga studios and gyms are very different environments, teachers often treat them the same. But people who patronize yoga studios are generally ready to get deeper into yoga's philosophy and Hindu trappings. They expect the statues and chants and harmonium and Tibetan bowls. Many gym goers are simply looking for more flexible hamstrings. Some come in skeptically, especially guys dragged in by their female partners, and are looking for proof that yoga *isn't* for them. One even turned up in my class because he lost a Super Bowl bet.

As for my background, I was born Catholic. I've been interested in the Hindu gods ever since meeting Hare Krishnas when I was 16. I've read a fair amount of yoga philosophy and have reflected upon it at length. Like many yoga teachers, I went through a phase of thinking I was a quasi-Hindu. But eventually I accepted that I am not and will never be a Hindu.

What's more, Hinduism is not a proselytizing religion; the Hindus don't want me. My spiritual makeup is a hybrid of Catholicism/yoga philosophy/12 step/agnosticism.

No problem. Yoga philosophy is available to any interested parties, regardless of religion or lack thereof. It's important to me that I let my students know there's more to yoga than just the poses. It doesn't matter whether they pursue the philosophy and/or believe it; that's their business. But I feel like I'm not doing my job if I ignore the ethical underpinnings and the many potentially helpful concepts that can alleviate suffering.

However, I'm not that good at talking extemporaneously about the yogic concepts. So I thought I'd find a basic book and read to my students during savasana. That was harder than I expected. There are a ton of yoga books on the market, many wonderful, but none fit my needs: short, stand-alone readings lasting one to three minutes that covered yoga philosophy in accessible language and demonstrated how the concepts related to the life of the modern gym yogi. Also, a lot of books assume that the readers agree with the writer and are already totally sold on yoga and on Hinduism. Some also ignore science or blur the lines between evidence and faith. I'm not anti-faith, but when presenting to a group of people with widely ranging beliefs, I think it's important to state, "this is what some people believe," or, "this is what I believe," not "this is the way it is." That's guaranteed to turn off a room full of intelligent adults.

I found one book that had many suitable passages. So *Happy Yoga* by Steve Ross became our Sunday class' textbook. For ten years. I don't know how many times I read the book through, a page at a time, week after week, skipping parts nobody wanted to hear, such as what Ross thought they should and shouldn't eat. I highly recommend *Happy Yoga*. But after ten years I was so sick of it I couldn't bear to drag it to class another week.

Again I went to the bookstore. Again I didn't find quite the book I was looking for.

I guess it's pretty predictable what happened next. I decided to write *Meditations for Gym Yogis*. I never really expected to write a yoga book. Looking at the shelves of Powell's, my local bookstore here in Portland, Oregon, it doesn't seem like the world could possibly need another yoga book. But there seemed to be a gap. And after more than a decade of teaching gym yogis, I aimed to fill it.

My book is based on reading I've done and classes and lectures I've attended as filtered through my own experience of life, spiritual practices and yoga. I hope you'll do the same, and filter everything you read about yoga through your own experience. And I hope you'll find this book useful, interesting and accessible. Thanks for picking it up.

WHAT IS YOGA AND WHAT'S IT FOR?

People have a lot of ideas about what yoga is and what it's for. Some worry it's a religion that will conflict with their own. Others view it as a means to attain the yoga butt. Many think it's solely about flexibility.

Yoga means "union," from the word "yuj," which is an oxen yoke, the thing that attaches the ox to the wagon. So what are you trying to attach to what? The idea is that you attach your own little self to the infinite.

Most people have probably experienced both an intense sense of separation, and a profound connection, at different times. Some days, my life feels like I'm a lone ant pushing something heavy over a steep and dirty curb. Other people, with their calls, demands and emails, hinder me. I suspect their motives and judge their character. Inanimate objects incur my wrath. It's an emotional place of isolation and often resentment and self-pity.

On other days, a simple walk in the neighborhood is a source of joy. I see shared humanity in my mailman, a neighbor, somebody pushing a shopping cart. I pet cats, admire flowers and feel that the same life animates all of us. The sky and ground are alive to me.

When I feel connected to the world around me, I'm 100 times happier.

Yoga is a system of practices – not a religion – by which you can dissolve the fears and self-consciousness that make you feel separate. But this process takes time, commitment and discipline. A lot of the practice is forming good habits: taking care of the body by doing postures that keep it strong and supple, whether you're in the mood or not. Treating others ethically, even when lying, cheating or evasion is more convenient. Learning to sit still and concentrate on the breath, which is by turns comforting and duller than dirt. These practices, and many more we'll discuss later, give us the foundation that will build toward enlightenment. Or at least bring a little peace, contentment and a more sustained feeling of connection.

TYPES OF YOGA

If you're new to the world of yoga classes, the different offerings are confusing. My own practice began in 1992, while I was on an extended trip through Asia. People stared when I jogged through the crowded streets. Desperate for exercise, I found a yoga book in a used bookstore. It was from 1969. I dutifully followed directions and consulted pictures of a skinny model in a leotard with ironed hair and frosted lipstick. Then I settled in San Francisco just down the street from a business calling itself the Yoga College of India. That sounded official. I took my first classes there. Men in Speedos and women in bikini tops did a repetitive sequence of poses in a carpeted studio heated to 105 degrees. Okay, so this was yoga, I thought. I practiced at home in a bikini top in front of the wall heater, much to my roommate's amusement. Later I went to classes strictly focused on alignment, then classes where we moved incessantly from pose to pose, then classes where we stretched out on bolsters and stayed as still as lizards. And these were just variations of hatha yoga, a catch-all term for the physical sorts of yoga favored by westerners.

In India, the birthplace of yoga, sages and seekers have come up with many types of yoga, all aimed at the goal of merging with the infinite. Most have nothing to do with physical postures. All are ways to dissolve the ego – the sense of a separate self – and merge with something greater. Often people with a particular bent choose a corresponding path. We'll just look at a few options, though there are more.

Karma yoga is the yoga of action. People who follow this path attempt to work selflessly, dedicating the results to the divine. The idea is that you work hard, doing the best you can for the world because it is your duty, but expecting nothing in return.

Spiritual brainiacs might choose jnana yoga, which involves lots of philosophical study and mental discipline. This is the path of wisdom and knowledge.

Bhakti yoga is all about love and devotion. Emotional people who enjoy prayer, singing and self-surrender are suited to bhakti yoga.

Raja, or "royal" yoga, involves mental, spiritual and physical aspects. A person practices eight activities that lead toward enlightenment. Of these, the third is asana, the postures we do in class. So the postures are only one-eighth of raja yoga. The other parts, which we'll explore later, are ethical principles, withdrawal of the senses, concentration, meditation and the final goal of merging with the divine.

YOGA SUTRAS: THE BIBLE OF YOGA

The text from which modern yoga eventually sprang was written about 2,000 years ago by Patanjali, an Indian sage. The Yoga Sutras is a collection of aphorisms that explain how to use yoga for spiritual development. Physical postures are barely mentioned. The Yoga Sutras focus on ethics, meditation, developing one-pointed concentration and, eventually, enlightenment.

Many books of commentary have been published on Patanjali's work. The 196 sutras, if printed alone, would fill less than 10 pages. But yogic scholars have unpacked the aphorisms for readers. Each sutra is only a line or two. The explication might go on for pages.

The writer of the Yoga Sutras may or may not have been the same Patanjali who was a noted Indian grammarian. I absolutely love his birth story, though it's not the sort of tale our western minds are likely to take seriously.

Here goes: Patanjali was an incarnation of Adidesa, the multi-headed cosmic serpent upon whom the god Vishnu rests. Vishnu predicted that the god Shiva would bless Adidesa with the chance to incarnate as a human, write a grammar book and master the art of dancing. In Adidesa's meditation, he began to search for a suitable mother through which to incarnate. He found Gonika, an older woman and yoga expert who had always yearned for a son. She figured her time for motherhood had passed, but made one last prayer to the sun god. She scooped up some water as an oblation. When she opened her hands, she saw a tiny snake. It changed into a tiny baby: her son, Patanjali.

The Yoga Sutras is *the* important yoga book and is oft-quoted in yoga studios. The ethical precepts Patanjali set forth, his strategies for minimizing the suffering in life, and much of his advice is timeless. We'll check in with what Patanjali has to say about yoga philosophy in the upcoming sections.

Perhaps the most famous sutra, and the one the average yoga teacher is most likely to be able to quote in Sanskrit, is "Yogah cittavritti nirodhah." It translates to, "Yoga is the cessation of fluctuations of the mind." So Patanjali is saying that through the practices detailed in his book, you can learn to quiet the mind. This promise is welcome news, as many people seek a break from minds that run 24/7. The next two sutras are "Then, the seer dwells in his own true splendor" and "At other times, the seer identifies with his fluctuating consciousness." Here, the seer is that timeless, eternal part of us that's linked to the soul.

5

These three little sutras sum up the problem and the solution. The goal of yoga is to help us dwell in our true splendor, rather than to be distracted by the fluctuations of consciousness, which revolve around thoughts, things, desires and aversions. Patanjali says that a quiet mind, with the seer in control, will bring peace, contentment and, eventually, enlightenment.

AHIMSA: NONVIOLENCE

The path of raja, or royal, yoga involves eight limbs. The first is a series of ethical restraints, called yamas. These five restraints improve characters and personalities, making it easier for people to live with each other.

Ahimsa is the first of the five yamas. "Himsa" means violence in Sanskrit, and the prefix "a" means without. So, nonviolence.

At first, this one might seem easy. Many of us might not think we need to work on nonviolence. Maybe we're anti-gun. We don't get in bar brawls or kick the dog. We might never even curse other drivers or give them the finger.

But look deeper.

Mahatma Gandhi, that paragon of nonviolence, had a lot to say about the nuances of ahimsa. "Ahimsa does not simply mean non-killing," he said. "Ahimsa means not to injure any creature by thought, word or deed. True ahimsa should mean a complete freedom from ill-will and anger and hate and an overflowing love for all."

Uh oh. How overflowing is your love? How free are you from ill will?

Unfortunately, I often catch myself having unlovely and unfair thoughts about other people. How do I know that another driver is an idiot who shouldn't be allowed on the road? Maybe I should give them the benefit of doubt. A bee could have snuck into their car and stung them, accounting for erratic driving. And did I really have a completely unfair flash of dislike for that young woman, just because she looks great in skinny jeans?

People are often harshest with themselves. What is that little voice saying in your head? If you catch yourself thinking you're not good enough, not attractive enough, not bright enough – or, with super-sized himsa, outright calling yourself bad, ugly or stupid – well, aren't you injuring yourself by thought?

If you're just starting to work on ahimsa, you can think of it as a three-step process of deed, word and thought which you're refining. First, you learn to not kick the dog. Second, you refrain from saying to the dog, "I could just kick you!" And third, you stop even thinking about kicking the dog. Now you're well on the road to perfecting ahimsa.

SATYA: TELL THE TRUTH

The second of the moral restraints, or yamas, is satya, which means truth. We're supposed to tell the truth. So does this mean going around venting freely, giving voice to every thought, with no filter between lips and mind? No. Notice that satya falls under the list of restraints. This means speaking the truth, but carefully.

When I contemplate satya, it makes me think of the ninth step in 12-step programs. In this step, people make amends to those they have harmed except when doing so would injure them or others. Giving thought to injury is key. Often people convince themselves that they're telling somebody something because it's right to tell the truth. After they tell their truth they feel free and don't even notice they have simply transferred the burden to their confidante. Instead, satya would have you bear the burdens that are yours to bear and spare the innocents around you. This, of course, goes with the first yama, ahimsa. What good is telling the truth if it results in harming the person you tell?

Satya also brings up the problem of what is truth? While such a thing as absolute truth may or may not exist, neither you nor I have a handle on it. At any given time, what we believe is true is a cocktail of information and emotions filtered through our own experience. This means that each person will have her own perspective.

I once had a boyfriend who believed he was privy to absolute truth. He frequently prefaced his sentences with "The reality of the situation is," or "At the end of the day." Then he'd try to pass off his opinion as truth. This approach was alienating, because it left no room for other people's perspectives. In other words, it made me want to scream. And I might as well have, since cornering the market on truth renders other people's words useless.

When contemplating how to improve communication, consider master yogi BKS Iyengar's counsel. He divides poor use of speech into four categories: abuse and obscenity, dealing in falsehoods, telling tales and ridiculing what others hold sacred.

ASTEYA: NO STEALING

Have you ever not picked up your phone because you knew it was a friend calling to complain for the hundredth time about her relationship woes? Or, worse, have you realized that people were screening their calls to avoid *your* repetitive saga?

This kind of time suck is a subtle aspect of asteya, the third of the yamas, or moral restraints of yoga. "Steya" means stealing and "a" means not. So this yama tells us not to steal.

Asteya may look easy at first. Assuming you're not a thief, you might think you have it made. Maybe you've never stolen a material object in your life. Even former juvenile delinquents might say to themselves, "Well, I've got that one covered. Gave up shoplifting at 15."

But there are other ways to steal, including leaning too hard on people for their time and energy.

In the situation mentioned above, you might answer the call from your lovesick friend. After listening to an hour-long rant, your friend says, "I always feel so much better after talking to you." But you don't. You feel like you've been sucked dry by an energy vampire. This friend is stealing your emotional energy as well as your time.

If you recognize *yourself* in the description of this friend, perhaps you could be kinder to your confidantes. Work through your problems in a journal or support group or with a competent counselor.

People also take from each other by overusing somebody's skills. It's lovely to help others out and to accept their help. But if you assume that every weekend your friend should snake your drains, clean your gutters, update your websites, hem your pants, or otherwise donate all their spare hours to you, it's time to learn to do these tasks yourself or pay somebody for their labor. Parents who work at home, self-employed people or anybody else with a flexible schedule are particular targets of time thieves.

Asteya also involves not taking what is not freely offered. If you nag people for favors, those favors are not being freely offered. When you steal what's not yours, usually you're operating from a place of lack or a place of entitlement. Neither is a pretty place.

To make sure you're not stealing, consider whether you're doing your fair share in your relationships. Everybody faces occasional hardships and needs some extra TLC. But over time, try to strike an approximate balance.

BRAHMACHARYA: SEXUAL VIRTUE

I once went to a party where some of the guests knew the host from a polyamorous group. Being a friendly person, I unknowingly engaged one of these men in conversation and accidentally gave him the impression I, too, was some kind of swinger. For the rest of the night, he shadowed me. Every time I looked up from a conversation with another guest, he leered at me from nearby as though I were a juicy steak. Not surprisingly, this sex vibe gave me the creeps. It seemed like his interactions were distilled down to one aspect of life, like a one-dimensional cartoon character, making him both laughable and sad.

When you focus only on sex – or other compulsive behaviors – sooner or later it narrows your world-view and depletes you. You may neglect your health, work, other interests and emotional and spiritual wellbeing.

That's why the fourth moral restraint of yoga is brahmacharya. This word comes from the god Brahman, Hinduism's eternal supreme godhead, and charya, or "to follow." So people who adhere to brahmacharya are living virtuous lives.

What comes as a shock to many Western yoga students is that traditionally, brahmacharya means celibacy. But like many aspects of yoga, brahmacharya has been reinterpreted and toned down for a modern western audience. Otherwise, yoga studios would be empty.

A more moderate view of brahmacharya is to discipline the use of sexual energy. Remember that the point of yoga is to transcend suffering caused by attachments, aversions and desires, so that you may work toward freedom from your limited, individual ego. In the Yoga Sutras, Patanjali, the great-granddaddy of yoga philosophy, stated that practicing brahmacharya results in unbounded vitality and energy.

Celibacy – or even moderation in sex and romance – may never catch on in the west. But it's worth considering. How much time do people you know spend on the internet, looking for instant sexual gratification on porn sites or future sexual gratification on dating sites? Is it possible that this time and energy could be better spent? How many opportunities are lost when you evaluate each person solely as a sexual conquest?

In modern times, brahmacharya is often defined as "sexual continence." Depending on your situation, this could mean celibacy, fidelity to a partner or, at the very least, honesty in your sexual dealings rather than sneaking around. Dishonest sex relations squander a great deal of psychic and emotional energy. Plus they violate the first yama, ahimsa, or nonharming.

Some modern yogis also interpret brahmacharya as moderation and apply the concept to all those things people tend to go a little crazy over: drinking to excess, overeating, shopping, video games, gambling, watching TV or anything else that diverts a great deal of your time, energy, money and mental space away from more productive and genuinely fulfilling uses.

APARIGRAHAHA: NON-HOARDING

In recent years, hoarding has come into the public consciousness. TV shows enter the hoarder's lair, revealing staggering heaps of junk. In my state of Oregon, a hoarder recently got into trouble with her hoarding niche: more than 100 orange cats. Hoarding has sparked the public's imagination as a bizarre mental health issue. Yoga questions the morality of hoarding.

Aparigraha is yoga's fifth yama, or moral restraint. "Parigraha" means to hoard or collect. The prefix "a" means not. So aparigraha is the opposite of hoarding. The idea here is to not fill your home and life with a whole bunch of stuff you don't need in the foreseeable future.

Even if you don't stack newspapers to your ceiling or keep dozens of mangy felines, hoarding can show up in subtler ways. I'm afraid I'm familiar with this one, as demonstrated by weird quirks like holding onto the last little bit of something in a bottle when it should be thrown away, or rushing to look in free boxes when there's really nothing I need. Nobody could say I require more pairs of black yoga pants than I already have, but then I see a really cute pair on sale and can't seem to pass them up. Maybe parigraha shows up in your life as a sentimental attachment to too many old objects, or a basement full of appliances that don't work but could possibly be fixed one day.

One argument against this accumulation of material possessions is that it weighs you down and ties you to the material world. You worry about where to put your stuff, how to maintain your stuff, or what will happen when it's lost or damaged. People may stay in harmful and unhappy situations because they feel trapped in a lifestyle full of material possessions. How many miserable couples stay together because they can't figure out how to divide their stuff?

Hoarding also shows a lack of faith. Depending on your philosophy, do you not trust in God, the universe or yourself to supply your material needs next year or a decade from now?

I'm not suggesting you shouldn't own things or care about your belongings. You just shouldn't care so much about things that they rule your life. And if you are operating from a deep sense of lack, it's time to stop and examine that and reassure yourself that you do, indeed, have enough. That you are enough.

SAUCHA: CLEANLINESS

Every year, one of my New Year's resolutions is to be tidier. I'm better than I used to be, but it's a long slow road. I tend to read several books at a time, and be in the midst of multiple writing and art projects. One of my college roommates used to call the assortment of papers and art supplies around my preferred end of the couch "Lake Teresa." Many years later, I've made the modest improvement of moving my lake to a table rather than the living room floor.

Unfortunately for me, cleanliness is one of the mandates of yoga.

The five yamas, or moral restraints – things yogis aren't supposed to do – compose the first limb of yoga. The second limb is made of five things yogis *are* supposed to do. These are called niyamas. Taken together, there are a total of ten yamas and niyamas. Yogis who come from Christian traditions sometimes liken them to the ten commandments.

The first niyama, saucha, means cleanliness or purity, and has both external and internal manifestations. The most obvious is how you keep the space around you. Is your house clean and tidy? Are your dust bunnies the size of raccoons? Do you arrange your yoga props neatly behind your mat? Or do blocks, straps and discarded socks ring your mat unevenly?

Then there's cleanliness of the body. Many people have had the unpleasant experience of practicing yoga next to a student who thinks yoga's goal of liberation includes freedom from showering and deodorant. Nope. Saucha tells you to clean your body before going to yoga. Or anywhere.

Going internal and getting more personal. What do you eat? Nutritious food or junk? Saucha encourages you to treat your body as a temple and to eat what will nourish rather than sicken you over time.

And now, even more personal. What are you thinking? Are you constantly judging or categorizing yourself and others? Do you allow your mind to be consumed by resentments, guilt, self-pity and pettiness? Sure, you can't help it if ugly thoughts enter your mind. But do you really need to devote your life to gnawing on them? This is where a yoga or meditation practice can help to redirect your thoughts and thus clean up your mind.

How do you redirect your mind? By catching it in the act. Sometimes I catch myself feeling a vague crankiness or anger and I don't even know why. I have to slow down and try to perceive its source. Usually it's an ugly thought just barely in my consciousness. When you can still the mind enough to root out these thoughts, you can redirect them by thinking of something more productive, or directing your attention away from thought by focusing on your breathing, a mantra or sensations in your body.

SANTOSHA: THE PURSUIT OF CONTENTMENT

Do you ever ruin your day by dwelling on your extra 15 pounds, middle-aged jowls, ugly house, stupid partner or ungrateful kids? Or by coveting your friend's job, perfect figure, talents, better looking partner or fat bank account?

Yoga's second niyama, or moral imperative, is santosha. This translates from Sanskrit as "contentment." To be your happiest, you must cultivate contentment. That means appreciating what you have in your life right now, rather than wasting energy despairing that your life isn't different. Yogis avoid envying others. They also try not to lament former versions of themselves, whether younger, thinner, healthier or in happier relationships. Contentment means you are already satisfied and are thus free of desires.

It's impossible to accurately compare your insides with other people's outsides. You know what you're feeling, but you have no idea what is really going on with somebody else. This point has been driven home to me several times, most notably by a yoga student. While I was teaching at a yoga studio, a handsome young man attended classes there for a month or so. I didn't give him much thought, except to notice his good looks and friendliness. If I'd had to guess, I would have said he was a happy, popular fellow with a relatively easy life.

But one day the studio received a letter from him. He revealed that he had come to the studio at a low point. In fact, he was contemplating suicide. The letter thanked the studio's teachers for giving him enough hope and enough good feelings to not kill himself. Wow. I've pondered this letter so many times. It presents multiple lessons. One is to never underestimate the effect your everyday interactions can have on the people around you. I had no idea he was in a fragile state. What if I'd had a bad day and snapped at him? As far as santosha, this guy seemed eminently covetable: young, handsome, apparently healthy, with probably no trouble finding a date. Yet inside he hurt so badly he wanted to die. This reminded me that I should never assume anybody has it easy. I need to make peace with my own lot in life, not wish I had somebody else's.

So how do you become content? For some people, it's easier than others. You might be naturally optimistic. If you're not, you'll need to work harder to cultivate a positive perspective and to be grateful for what you have. Of course, it's easier to do this kind of psycho-spiritual work when your basic needs of food, shelter and healthcare are met. But don't assume that richer equals more contentment. Just look at all the drama in the lives of celebrities.

Santosha does not mean that you shouldn't try to change your lot in life. If you're in a dangerous or abusive situation, or suffering from addiction, changing that is a priority. You need to take whatever steps are necessary to get safer and healthier. But you can still cultivate contentment along the way. Maybe you'll be in rehab, a domestic violence shelter or a small and ugly apartment until you get back on your feet. Enjoy your progress. Try to focus on lessons learned rather than time wasted. While somebody else built a fortune in real estate, maybe you built a fortune in empathy and experience you can share with others who are going through the same struggles. There's value – and a reason to find contentment – in so many situations.

SVADHYAYA: STUDYING YOURSELF AND SACRED TEXTS

Some people find themselves absolutely fascinating. They'll enjoy part of the fourth niyama, or ethical imperative, of yoga. Svadhyaya calls for both study of the self and studying sacred texts.

Studying ourselves takes a certain amount of detachment. If you've been in therapy, 12-step groups or are naturally self-reflective, you are probably already familiar with this concept. Instead of just going through life reacting to external stimuli, you stop and think about your behavior. Are you acting fairly? Are you being kind? Are you letting yourself be triggered by predictable stimuli and then blaming someone else for it? When your partner acts heinously, what's your part in the mess?

The study of spiritual texts might be harder, since they're not exactly page-turners. Yoga comes from Hinduism, so yogis have traditionally studied sacred texts such as the Vedas. This large body of ancient scriptures is written in Sanskrit and dates back as far as 1500 B.C. Some modern western yogis enjoy reading the Vedas in translation or, for a few intrepid scholars, in the original language. The Bhagavad Gita is pretty accessible, especially the editions with explanatory notes.

But it's not necessary to become a pseudo-Hindu to do yoga. I've seen many yoga students and teachers get absolutely rapturous about anything Hindu, whether they understand the words or not. While it's great to appreciate other people's religion, some of these rapturous folks cut Hinduism all kinds of slack yet turn a critical or even contemptuous eye toward the religion of their youth.

The Dalai Lama —who is a Buddhist, not a Hindu – encourages seekers not to be swept away by foreignness and exoticism, but to give their native religion a close look. He says, "I always tell my Western friends that it is best to keep your own tradition. Changing religion is not easy and sometimes causes confusion. You must value your tradition and honor your own religion."

In this spirit, perhaps svadhyaya for you means checking out the texts of your Jewish, Wiccan, Christian, Muslim or whatever roots. And if you're opposed to religion, you could read some inspirational poetry. At the very least, do the self-study part of this niyama so you bring a more self-reflective presence to the world.

TAPAS: SPIRITUAL ZEAL

Most people are familiar with burning zeal in one way or another. This same sort of tireless energy can take a gazillion different forms. Olympic athletes, politicians, people who picket abortion clinics, scientists bent on cures, anorexics, Black Friday shoppers and gamers who play the same game for 20 hours straight all demonstrate burning zeal for varying goals. Tapas, yoga's third niyama, or ethical mandate, is about harnessing that energy for spiritual practice. It refers to directing your greatest energy into your spiritual life.

Saints from all religions have done this for ages. I recently visited the shrine of Santa Narcisa de Jesus in Ecuador and was impressed to learn of her busy tapas-driven schedule: eight hours a day of praying, followed by four evening hours of self-flagellation. Some yogis, especially the holy men and women of India, follow similarly hardcore regimens. Some stand on one leg for years, surviving on only two glasses of milk per day.

But the modern gym yogi can take a more low-key approach to tapas. Remember that the goal of yoga is to end suffering. People usually go to the gym because they want better health and the better life that brings. But there might be days you would rather do something other than take care of your body. Many times I arrive at the community center where I take classes and it occurs to me hey, I could skip boot camp and just get lunch or stop by Target and look at the clearance rack. Tapas means I acknowledge that thought but don't let it derail my commitment to health and fitness. I get out of the car, enter the building and participate to the best of my ability.

In addition to bringing tapas to your physical movements, you can apply this principle to meditation. Same with any prayer or spiritual reading you do. You can find that burning zeal for the worthwhile things you are doing, and keep at them.

But remember to temper tapas with compassion. It's easy to use this sort of energy for bad ends. Many gym-goers get obsessed with the physical body to the point that eating disorders and/or injuries ensue. It's a waste of energy to direct all your zeal into perfecting your body; eventually it will grow old and die. Save some zeal for your spirit. Yoga teacher Rolf Gates emphasizes the need to ground tapas in gratitude for what you have, a sense of wonder about what the world offers, and respect for others. Tapas is internal, not something to show off. Don't try to compare your tapas to the level of zeal that others have for their practice.

ISVARA PRANIDHANA: SURRENDER TO GOD

Many religions involve surrendering your own will to a bigger picture. Christian prayers include wording like, "Thy will, not mine, be done." Spiritual seekers often acknowledge that they had one plan for their lives, but then circumstances took them in a much different direction, which they attributed to the will of God.

The fifth niyama, or moral imperative of yoga, is isvara pranidhana, which means surrender to God. If you're religious, this is easy to understand, but probably still not easy to do. If you're agnostic, this concept will seem pretty vague. If you're an atheist, reading this might annoy you.

If you do have a concept of God, Source, spirit, or whatever you want to call it, you can think of your yoga postures, your job, things you do for others, your creative work and hobbies, all dedicated to and feeding into this great power for good. When your life takes sudden, unexpected turns, you try to see it as God's will.

Some anti-religion folks find themselves in situations where they're strongly encouraged to acknowledge and adopt a higher power. This happens all the time in 12-step groups, and is probably the biggest sticking point. Step three states, "Made a decision to turn our will and our lives over to the care of God as we understood him." People who don't believe in a sentient higher power face a real challenge getting to the other nine steps if they're stuck on three. So members of anonymous groups come up with workarounds. Some state that GOD stands for Good Orderly Direction, and that following a plan like the 12 steps can be a higher power than they have on their own. Others acknowledge that the collective wisdom of the group is greater than their own limited resources, and consider the group their higher power. Part of the point is admitting that many things are beyond a single human's control, and recognizing that there are big forces you can choose to align yourself with or not.

Some yogis will never embrace this niyama. My own concepts around a higher power are pretty fuzzy. I think of God as a big mystery beyond human comprehension. All the religions are human-created lenses that try to understand something out of reach. I embrace the simplest lessons in and out of church about being a good person, and tend to disregard the rest. My priest speaks English as a second language, which keeps his sermons simple and focused. He often returns to the acronym JOY. Love Jesus (or fill in the blank with your higher power), Others and Yourself. Simple and easy to remember.

I'm not convinced God has such a specific plan for me that I should just sit on the couch and wait for it to unfold. So I make the best plans I can. But occasionally it seems like big forces are at play and maybe some mystical stuff is happening that I don't comprehend. And it might even be to my benefit.

Whatever. Everybody will have an easier time with some of these concepts than with others. And the ones that confuse you more will just be works in progress for years or for your entire lifetime. That's okay. You don't have to do this all perfectly.

ASANA: YOGA POSTURES

Asana is the third of the eight limbs of yoga. This is by far the best known in the western world. Asana translates from Sanskrit as "comfortable seat," but is generally interpreted as postures. Warrior one, child's pose and downward dog are all examples of common asanas.

The original aim of doing all these postures was to make the body strong and healthy enough to sit in long periods of meditation. While using asana to prepare for meditation is still terrific, many modern yogis use the postures to counteract long periods of sitting at a computer or in a car.

I've heard many yoga and spiritual teachers admonish students that they absolutely must make time to meditate. If everybody spent time meditating, we'd probably have a more ideal and less stressed world. But too often I find that not meditating becomes another source of guilt, another thing on the to-do list like cleaning the gutters, organizing the spice rack and learning a second language.

For many gym yogis, asana may be as close to meditation as they ever come. And that's okay. Asana works as a moving meditation. The key is integrating the breath with the movements to keep you in the moment. In many ways, asana is easier than meditation because the physical effort and bodily sensations help anchor you in the present by giving your mind something to focus on.

When I ask a class which poses they like the best and least, it's always interesting to hear the difference of opinions. Favorite poses are frequently the ones that are easiest, that feel best, or, for students who have been practicing longer, the ones that used to be difficult but now are doable. Practicing asana parallels living our lives. Sometimes we struggle and want to give up. Sometimes it doesn't seem worth the effort. But by showing up and consistently practicing postures, we build our tenaciousness along with our strength.

The uncomfortable poses can be the most valuable. Practicing staying in the discomfort of poses has helped me in other areas of my life. I've had to lie still while a dermatologist cut skin cancers out of my face. I automatically started slowing the breath and stilling my body, just like I would in a difficult pose I was trying to stay in.

On the physical level, you can feel your muscles working or stretching, depending on the pose. At a subtler level, practicing asana helps move energy. Yogis believe there are 72,000 energy channels, called nadis, in your body. That's a lot of chances for a blockage! Asana keeps us open and running smoothly both physically and metaphysically.

PRANAYAMA: BREATH CONTROL

I once subbed a power yoga class where one of the students could not sit still and breathe for two minutes. While the other students sat quietly, she writhed as though being poked with sticks. After two minutes, she rolled up her mat, said "This isn't working for me," and left.

Some people seem proud that they can't sit still and breathe. They consider themselves too active, athletic, busy or smart to waste time this way. But what is sitting and breathing about? Control and mastery of the self.

In a way, everybody knows this. Even the least New Agey people might admit there's merit in the classic advice about stopping, taking a deep breath and counting to ten before you hit somebody or say something you'll surely regret. This is an example of using the breath for self-mastery. Instead of being carried forward by the momentum of anger or hurt, you stop and practice being less reactive.

I suspect some of the people who are proud of themselves for having better things to do than breathe might actually be fearful of sitting still. Who would you be if you were quiet and not accomplishing things 24/7? If there was nobody to text? What would you hear inside the mind with your TV, phone and iPod shut off?

Learning to control the breath is pranayama, the fourth limb of yoga. A variety of exercises fall into this category, such as ujaiya breath, breath of fire, skull polishing breath and alternate nostril breathing. Each has a different physical and metaphysical function. But each is ultimately a way of mastering yourself.

Think about breathing. All day you do it unconsciously. Just as you generally do other things unconsciously, including thinking and feeling. Moods and attitudes are constantly swayed by thoughts and feelings people seldom take the time and self-awareness to decipher. So you can look at breathing as a symbol of all your unconscious acts. All have consequences which you'll have to live with. Once you understand that breathing can be used to slow down, stay in the moment, change your mood and avoid regrettable behavior, you're on the road to finding other ways to avoid knee-jerk reactions to external stimuli.

PRATYAHARA: WITHDRAWAL OF THE SENSES

When I studied with yoga teacher Todd Williamson, he sometimes had us do an exercise where we'd lie with our eyes closed and pretend we were at the bottom of a deep ocean. Very far above us, we knew waves broke the surface of the sea. But we could see or hear nothing. It was dark at the bottom of the ocean, and peaceful, and we felt far from all the small fluctuations and turbulence of our sensory-driven lives. This is the feeling of pratyahara, the fifth limb of yoga.

Because the point of yoga is to transcend all the fluctuations of the mind and mood caused by external stimuli, pratyahara is about withdrawing the senses. What you see, hear, taste, smell and touch are all manifestations of the temporal world. If you want to go beyond the impermanent, you have to cultivate detachment from your senses.

This doesn't mean that you shouldn't appreciate sights, sounds, tastes and smells. But spending time withdrawing from stimuli helps to separate the material from the spiritual. You can still appreciate listening to a favorite song or eating a cookie, but are reminded that there are bigger things to organize your life around.

So how do you withdraw the senses? Meditation is one way. When you sit still and close your eyes in a quiet place, you minimize most of the senses. A more dramatic way is to spend time in a flotation tank.

But you can also practice in small ways. You can try closing your eyes in yoga poses you're most familiar with. Do savasana with an eye pillow over your eyes and earplugs in your ears. Spend time in your house or car without the stimulus of music or television. If your impulse is to snack when stressed, distracting yourself with taste and chewing, don't.

As you take breaks from fleeting sensory perceptions, you'll increase your awareness of deeper parts of yourself that are usually obscured by noise and sights.

DHARANA: ONE-POINTED CONCENTRATION

If you've sat around a dinner table where everybody is simultaneously texting, checking emails, eating and talking to their dinner companions, you know how rare one-pointed concentration is these days. But this old-fashioned concept is the sixth limb of yoga.

By practicing postures, breath control and withdrawal of the senses, you prepare the mind for dharana, one-pointed concentration. All your energy and attention is on the task you're doing in the present moment.

When you start to work on this, your mind will at first be wild, constantly jumping between subjects, unable to focus on one for more than a matter of seconds. As you practice stilling the mind, your ability to focus slowly improves.

People who are able to focus their minds this intensely will be able to achieve a lot. They could use it to make money, find a cure for a disease, write books or master any desired skill. Dharana can make you powerful.

But for yogis and other spiritual seekers, the idea is to shine your one-pointed focus on God, as you would an industrial strength flashlight. Sometimes this is done by chanting Om, or repeating mantras. Other spiritual traditions use similar practices. For example, The Jesus Prayer is popular with Eastern Orthodox Catholics. While it has many variants, a common form of this prayer goes, "Lord Jesus Christ, Son of God, have mercy on me, the sinner." Sometimes it's shortened to just three words: "Jesus, have mercy." Just like yoga mantras, the Jesus Prayer is often repeated silently, synchronized with breathing. Many monks repeat the Jesus Prayer incessantly, internalizing the prayer until they believe they are praying unceasingly, even while sleeping. This is an impressive example of dharana.

To start practicing concentration, close your eyes and conjure up an image. I like to focus on the Hindu god Shiva seated in meditation, since he concentrates so well. You could focus on Jesus or any conception of God. Or keep it secular by focusing on a common object like an apple. Whatever you choose, picture it as clearly as possible and try to keep all your attention fixed on it. This will be difficult at first, as your mind will want to dredge up memories and worries, and create conversations with people who aren't here. Go back to the god or the apple. With practice, concentrating will become much easier.

DHYANA: MEDITATION

The fifth and sixth limbs of yoga are dharana and dhyana, which are similar in both name and activity. Dharana is intense concentration. Dhyana is meditation. These two can be hard to differentiate. Where does concentration end and meditation start?

Yoga teacher Judith Lassater uses a water analogy to better understand this difference. She says when it's raining, you can feel the individual drops. But when you encounter a river, you can't tell one drop of water from another. They merge into a constant flow.

Concentration is like drops of rain. There are lapses in your concentration. Meditation is like the unceasing river.

Of course, this is the ideal. Most people don't have quiet minds. In fact, it might be really loud in there, with regrets, desires, insights and random memories all trying to shout each other down. When you sit to meditate, it helps to have very low expectations. Many people quit meditating because they say their minds are too busy, so they're no good at meditation. They seem to think everybody else has it easy. But truly, most people aren't good at meditation. Having a busy mind is the norm. And if clearing the mind was so easy, it wouldn't be worth practicing.

Instead, when you meditate – whether it's for two minutes at the beginning of yoga class or for half an hour at home – be gentle with yourself. Accept that thoughts arise. Sometimes a lot of thoughts. Try to observe them without engaging. Then go back to focusing on your breath or mantra or whatever you're using as a meditation tool. If the thoughts are persistent, you might have a thought and a mantra in your mind at the same time. That's okay. Try not to let the incessant thoughts frustrate you. It's a lot like an asana practice. You may not be able to reach our toes in a forward bend, but reaching in that direction stretches you. So do your imperfect attempts to meditate.

SAMADHI: MERGING WITH THE DIVINE

The last of the eight limbs of yoga, samadhi is when your consciousness merges with the divine. This is the same as the Buddhist concept of nirvana, except that nirvana is permanent and is usually reached after death of the physical body. Advanced yogis enter into this state of bliss during meditation while still alive.

This is one of those concepts that can feel very foreign to westerners. When Americans work hard at something, they generally expect a reward, whether it be money, fame, a trophy, heartfelt thanks or, at the very least, a feeling of accomplishment. That's not what samadhi promises. Instead, you get to be subsumed. Or liberated, depending on how you look at it.

Another contrast is that western civilization is heavily Christian. Americans are apt to believe in a personal god who takes great interest in people's struggles, from battling cancer to finding a parking space. While Hindus make offerings to various gods, the supreme god is pretty remote. It's not setting a place for you at the cosmic table and telling the angels to tune their harps for your welcome song.

When I was 24, I had a chance to travel in Indonesia. I visited Borobudur, an enormous ninth century Buddhist temple on the island of Java. The temple is built to demonstrate the stages of spiritual development people must go through to attain Buddhahood. Visitors circle around successively higher stone terraces lined with more than 600 stupas. A stupa is a structure shaped like a bell. Inside each stupa at Borobudur stands a Buddha statue.

It was hot and humid. Dripping sweat, I finally got to the very top level, to the central and largest stupa. After all that climbing, I expected to find the most impressive Buddha statue of all. But as I peered inside, I saw it was empty.

It was a little hard to wrap my mind around. I came from a culture and an era where the film "Rocky" made a big impression. Running up all those stairs led to a trophy, a title and a catchy theme song. But Buddhists and Hindus run up all those stairs to transcend.

After a couple of decades of reflection, some days I really see the appeal of permanently merging with the divine. Other days, I still want the trophy.

But don't worry. Most of us are in no imminent danger of reaching nirvana and permanently transcending our egos. However, glimpses of the divine are pretty sweet.

WHAT'S UP WITH OM?

The chanting of Om can divide yoga students. Some find it a meaningful and spiritual experience. Others consider it weird and not what they came for. This is especially true amongst gym yogis. While yoga studios often attract spiritual seekers, gyms are secular spaces. That's not to say that gym goers are less spiritual than anybody else; but when you signed your gym contract, you probably weren't signing up to chant.

Chanting Om can be especially offputting if you don't know what it means. The usual explanation is that it's the sound the universe makes. Some claim that it's a sound saints hear when they meditate. According to spiritual teacher Sri Sri Ravi Shankar, "In the Bible too, it is said, 'In the beginning there was a word and the word was with God and the word was God.' That is Om. There they don't say which word. The word is Om."

Since most people aren't saints, they aren't able to corroborate these facts by meditating and listening for sounds. Instead, this seems to be one of the many spiritual beliefs you can choose to accept on faith, or not.

Those who prefer complicated, many-layered explanations can delve deeper into Om. To start with, it can more precisely be spelled a-u-m. Often people chant aum distinctly, with four parts: the a, u, m, and a rest after the sound. Scholars attribute meanings to each part of the word, such as each letter representing one of three states of ordinary consciousness and the rest afterwards representing transcending consciousness.

Personally, I don't sit home and Om alone. I'm happy to chant Om when I'm taking somebody else's class, but it's not part of my own practice. So it would feel pretty phony for me to lead an Om chorus at the gym.

However, some of my yoga teacher friends feel differently. Kimberly Dark, who teaches in Hawaii, believes in the experiential benefits of Om, whether people know the meaning or not. She thinks people feel the Om vibrations through their whole body and enjoy a physical benefit. Florida-based teacher Jenny Gallagher has led students in Om chants in various unusual places, including classes taught at gyms, a public school and a Christian church. In her training, she learned that the throat is the first place to age and that the vibration of chanting or singing keeps the throat muscles in better shape. "In my mind, it doesn't matter if you chant Om or sing Happy Birthday," she told me. "I just remind my students to sing."

Like the other aspects of yoga, it's a very personal practice. You get to decide which parts to adopt and which to skip. If you're in class and the teacher starts chanting, you can always opt out and just listen. Many people do feel a strong connection to the sound of Om, and feel that chanting Om enhances their lives.

NAMASTE: SALUTING EACH OTHER

Some beginners feel perplexed at the end of yoga class when everybody brings their hands into prayer position, bows and says "namaste." This can seem downright cultlike at first. And if you practice a religion, you might be especially concerned about the implications of namaste. What does it mean and who are you bowing to?

The word "namaste" comes from the Sanskrit "nama," to bow, "as", which means I, and "te," or you. So you're saying, "I bow you." Basically this means you bow to another. In yoga class, that's the teacher, though you can also bow to the other students. Hindus believe that everybody has the divine within her or him. Namaste symbolizes that the divine part of you, your soul, is recognizing and bowing to the other person's soul. You put your hands together in front of your heart because this divine spark is said to reside in the heart chakra.

I really love this idea. When I get caught up in my problems and mundane tasks, it's easy to see other people as obstacles that get in my way and interrupt my busy life. When I pause to recognize that other people hold the same divine spark I do, it's both humbling and egalitarian. We're each just a tiny piece of the divine big picture.

When performing namaste, slow down and have a moment of reverence for whatever lineage of teachers – yoga, parents, school, any kind of teachers – brought you to this moment. Remember your own spark of divinity, and that of others. It's easy to do namaste in a rote or perfunctory way, as the last thing that separates yoga class from checking the next thing off your list.

In India, namaste is used as both a greeting and a farewell. Often Indians bow without saying the word, as the word and meaning is implied in the gesture.

The idea of namaste can be useful in many situations outside of yoga class. You don't need to say it or even bow. Just think it. I use this idea all the time to try to overcome my impatience. When I'm running around town, trying to complete all my errands, it would be easy to blow off the people that make our modern conveniences possible. How many times have I seen a customer thrust money at a cashier, not even looking her in the eye, while talking on a phone? Instead, I'm inspired by my mother's example. Not only does she acknowledge the humanity of every worker in her usual haunts, she knows the names of their spouses, children and dogs. I try to keep this idea of divine spark meeting divine spark by looking each person in the eye and remembering we're all made of the same cosmic stuff. This enhances my most mundane trips to the gas station, market and bank. And it shifts me out of the ugly, impatient part of my nature.

CHAKRAS: ENERGY CENTERS

The word "chakra" is Sanskrit for disk. Sacred Hindu texts dating back 4,000 years refer to the chakras. These are energy centers in your body which some people believe can explain a lot about how you form patterns and do the things you do.

Chakras are not physical entities. They won't show up on an X-ray. You can't have a chakra transplant, no matter how you might long for one. The main seven chakras run along your spine, starting at the base and finishing just over the top of your head. They line up with major intersections of arteries, veins and nerves. Each corresponds to a different human need and desire, such as survival or sexuality. Chakras also correspond to development stages, colors, mantras and elements, among other things. The lowest chakras are identified with more primal desires. As you ascend through the seven chakras, the needs and desires become more subtle and more spiritual.

Chakra healing proponents say that people have too much of one chakra's energy and not enough of another, leading to psychological and physical imbalances. For example, too much energy at the heart chakra could make a person jealous, possessive or codependent, while too little could lead to loneliness and isolation.

It makes sense that thousands of years ago people would look for an organizing system like the chakras, before modern science discovered more about the human body. But even modern people who don't necessarily believe in these colorful wheels of energy can benefit from looking at actions and habitual patterns through the philosophical system of the chakras. We'll look at each of the seven main chakras individually in upcoming sections.

FIRST CHAKRA: THE ROOT AND SURVIVAL

The lowest of the seven main chakras is called muladhara, which means "root" in Sanskrit. It's located at the base of the spine. This chakra is all about survival, security and rooting into the earth. Without a healthy root chakra, you don't feel safe in the world.

According to psychologist Anodea Judith, who integrates chakra theory with western psychology, the first chakra develops between conception and your first birthday. So if your early childhood was insecure – for example if you suffered birth traumas or were neglected, malnourished or had difficulty bonding with your mother – you could face first chakra issues. Of course, you might not even know this, since memory doesn't start that early. First chakra issues can involve trust, food, health, prosperity and setting appropriate boundaries. They can manifest physically in intestinal and bowel disorders, problems with teeth, bones, legs and feet, or as eating disorders.

People with first chakra problems might feel disconnected from their bodies. When you feel disconnected, it's time to take care of yourself at a very basic level. You need to eat wholesome food, drink water, exercise and rest. Practices that bring you in touch with the earth will help this chakra. Walk barefoot. Dance, do yoga, run, lift weights. Massage and other kinds of touch can be healing. You need to reassure yourself that you're safe and have a right to exist.

SECOND CHAKRA: SWEETNESS AND SEX

While the first chakra is focused on survival and is therefore very self-oriented, the second chakra is about pleasure and connecting with others through emotion and sex.

The second chakra's Sanskrit name is svadhisthana, which means sweetness. It's located in the lower abdomen and is associated with the color orange. This chakra develops between the age of six months and two years. When it functions well, you have a healthy relationship with pleasure. When it's not in good shape, you experience extremes of frigidity and lack of emotion on one end, or sex addiction and constant emotional crises on the other. This chakra is also strongly associated with guilt.

Contemplating the chakras is hard because you're faced with all the things that have happened to make you the way you are. If you're raising children, you'll wonder if every little thing you do will affect your children's psyches. Some of the ways the second chakra is damaged include early sexual or emotional abuse, rejection, neglect, emotional manipulation, restriction of movement and austere religious upbringings that deny pleasure. Denying children's feelings also can lead to second chakra troubles.

Many sex and emotional problems are boundary issues. You might have such rigid, self-protective boundaries that you hide your emotions – even from yourself – and are sexually cold. On the other extreme, you may have no boundaries, sleeping around, sharing every feeling with anybody who will listen and constantly spinning out emotionally. Depending where you are on this spectrum, you may need to learn to relax your boundaries and let people in. Or you may need to learn to contain your emotions and not express every single feeling.

To heal yourself, you must acknowledge that you deserve pleasure, and that it's okay to have emotions and sexual impulses. But that you don't slavishly follow them everywhere.

THIRD CHAKRA: POWER!

The third chakra, located at the solar plexus – a dense area of nerves behind your stomach – is about power. Do you direct the course of your own life? Or are you the victim of circumstances? Depending on the availability of personal power stored in your third chakra, you may play the role of hero or martyr.

The name of the third chakra is manipura, which is Sanskrit for lustrous gem. It's associated with transformation, autonomy, will power, self-esteem, the color yellow and the element of fire. Too much energy in manipura makes you domineering, aggressive, arrogant, hyperactive and competitive. People with Type A personalities hold a lot of energy in their third chakras. Too little energy here and you may be easily manipulated, blame others for your troubles, lack self-esteem and self-discipline, and be passive and unreliable. Shame dwells in this chakra.

Psychologist and chakra expert Anodea Judith notes an interesting discrepancy between a healthy third chakra and many spiritual disciplines. Yoga and other spiritual paths aim to transcend the ego and merge with the divine. But having a healthy third chakra means you recognize yourself as an individual who determines your life's aims. You know what you're about, and you don't necessarily agree with everything your parents, spouse, friends or religion dictate.

Navigating between the spiritual and temporal worlds requires delicate balance. I like to think of tree pose here. You root down, the foot of your standing leg connected to the ground. At the same time, you reach toward the sky. With good posture your chakras form a perfect bridge through which you join the earthbound and heavenbound parts of yourself. It's beautiful to aspire toward heavenly merging. And it's beautiful to maintain enough power and sense of self to fulfill your earthly tasks. Which, if you want to live indoors and keep the lights on, probably requires enough self-will and determination to go out and earn a living. Pursuing meaning in your life also takes a substantial amount of grit and gumption. Both of which make their home in the third chakra.

FOURTH CHAKRA: THE UNSTRUCK HEART

I think the fourth chakra has the best name. Anahata is Sanskrit for "unstruck." This refers to the perfect state of the heart: not having been struck by any tragedy or grief. Probably nobody alive can honestly claim their heart has gone unstruck. But the name gives me hope that I can heal my heart back to some semblance of its unstruck state.

As you climb the chakras, they become more spiritually refined. So far we've gone from survival to sex to power and now to love. The anahata chakra is associated with the color green and the element of air. Its purpose is to love yourself and others. When it's balanced, you feel peace, compassion and empathy. A deficient heart chakra makes you judgmental, withdrawn, narcissistic and lonely. An excess of energy here leads to codependency, jealousy, clinging and a lack of boundaries.

Most people have felt a deficiency or an excess of love at some time. So how do you get an off-kilter anahata chakra back on-kilter? Sometimes it takes changing what you expect out of relationships. You might need to forgive yourself or others before you can truly trust and feel again. And while it's been said so much that it's a cliché, this bit of wisdom still holds true: You have to love yourself before you can love others. If you're in a state of self-loathing, you're sure to attract equally unhealthy characters. Often you need to learn to be alone and whole, to integrate the various parts of your personality and those traits that society deems masculine or feminine, before you're really suitable company for another healthy individual. When the anahata chakra is balanced, you complete yourself, rather than waiting for somebody else to do it for you.

FIFTH CHAKRA: SPEAK YOUR TRUTH

The fifth chakra, called visuddha, is located at the throat. So it's not surprising that this chakra is connected to communication and finding your voice. The neck is such a narrow structure, connecting the feeling body to the thinking head. This is an easy chakra to get jammed up.

Visuddha means purification. It's at this point in the chakras where you refine your impressions into speech. This is where you attempt to communicate your truth to others. Lies are the enemy of visuddha. The throat chakra is identified with sound, the color blue, creativity, symbolic thinking and self-expression.

If you lack energy in this chakra, you may fear speaking. And when you do speak up, your voice may be weak and breathy. You might lack the words for your feelings. Too much energy here and you're apt to talk too much and listen too little.

As with the other chakras, patterns form during childhood. If you kept secrets from a young age or heard lies, mixed messages or excessive criticism from your elders, you might develop problems with this chakra. And like the other chakras, the way to healing depends on whether you have too much or too little energy here. People who talk defensively, using a constant stream of conversation to avoid any real or deep communication, can practice silence and develop active listening skills. Those who haven't found their voices may benefit from singing, mantra, storytelling and neck and shoulder exercises. Each person brings a unique voice to the world. This is the chakra where you get the chance to share that special voice.

SIXTH CHAKRA: THE THIRD EYE

Just above and between your eyebrows is your third eye. This spiritual eye is often depicted vertically on Hindu statues. Many Hindus wear a bindi, a red dot or more ornate sticker, on their foreheads to represent the third eye. This is the site of the sixth chakra. Its Sanskrit name is ajna, which means to perceive and command. This is where the conscious and unconscious mind merge, the part of you that understands dreams, mythology and symbolism.

Ajna chakra is associated with light, the color indigo, self-reflection, memory, dream recall, clairvoyance and the ability to visualize. A balanced sixth chakra allows you to perceive bigger patterns and meanings in your life.

When ajna is deficient, you might be all about rational thought and no intuition. You miss social cues. You can't imagine how your life could be different. Instead, you accept that this is just how you are and there's no hope for change. This also makes you less empathetic. You may not remember your dreams.

Too much third eye energy is even more dangerous. An excess in the sixth chakra often corresponds with insufficient energy in lower chakras. This lack of grounding can result in huge, unrealistic dreams to the point of delusion. You may hallucinate and develop paranoia. If this is the case, focus on energizing your lower chakras.

To further develop ajna chakra, you need to cultivate the ability to see your life on the symbolic level. You can read mythology and contemplate the symbolic stories in the tales. To improve your dream recall, write down your dreams and share them with interested friends. Develop your intuition by listening to your gut instincts. Meditation also enhances the energy in ajna chakra.

SEVENTH CHAKRA: THE CROWN

The seventh chakra's Sanskrit name is sahasrara, which means thousandfold. It's often conceptualized as a thousand-petaled lotus. So you can imagine this is both a stunning and complex chakra.

Sahasrara is also called the crown chakra, and is located at or just above the crown of your head. When all the chakras are balanced and doing their part to make you a whole, creative, connected person, the energy flows up from your lower six chakras to your crown chakra and helps connect you to the divine. But it's a two-way street. Divinity also enters the crown chakra from above, flowing down into your body. Perhaps this is where songs and poems come from. With a balanced crown chakra, you connect with the infinite yet retain a home in the body

The crown chakra's mission is to derive meaning. This is where your belief structures – whether they be compiled from your personal experiences or forged by a particular religion or creed – dwell. If your sahasrara is balanced, your spiritual life expands as new information is integrated into your belief system. But if you're deficient here, cynicism may win out over spirituality, or you may have such rigid beliefs that you discount new information.

It's difficult as an adult living in the modern world to feel balanced in any of the chakras. And it's difficult for parents to bring up balanced children. Many people feel wounded by their spiritual upbringings. Some children of agnostic or atheist parents resent missing out on making early spiritual connections, or feel their spiritual yearnings are ridiculed by their families. And many children of religious parents resent having a rigid belief system stuffed down their throats.

One of my key religious memories is a nun insisting that Jesus had died for my particular sins. As an eight year-old who was born nearly 2000 years after those events transpired, this logic struck me as ludicrous. Not to mention that my first eight years yielded no sins worth dying over. I was so intellectually offended that it would be decades before I was even willing to consider the beauty and worthwhile lessons contained within my troubling childhood religion.

You might have memories that, like mine, jammed your crown chakra by derailing your belief systems. You may form reactionary belief systems, which you then filter your experiences through, rejecting any contradictory information. Instead, a healthy crown chakra requires you to loosen up, to allow your consciousness to expand and incorporate new ideas, and to develop your own concept of the divine that has meaning for you.

GUNAS: THREE CRUCIAL ELEMENTS

If you dig into yoga theory, you'll soon encounter the three gunas. A guna is a primordial element. Yogis say all matter and mental states are composed of these three elements in varying degrees. Just as three primary colors make up all the other colors and their many shadings, the gunas form your many moods, actions and thoughts.

Tamas is the state of inertia and stagnation. A tamasic person could be an inactive couch potato who's usually in a foul mood, eats lots of junk food and ignores their problems. Raja is about activity. A rajasic person is more active, drawn to spicy foods and caffeine, likes to get stuff done, blames others for their problems and might be spiritually lacking despite material success. The third guna, sattva, is about balance, purity and spiritual insight. This is the guna that yoga helps you work towards. Practicing yoga can bring more sattva into your life. If you feel calm and peaceful in yoga while doing relatively active poses, you're approaching the sattvic state.

So how do you use the gunas? If you want to come to a balanced place in your energy, you can check in with yourself and see how you are at any given movement. Depressed and can't get out of bed? That's an excess of tamasic energy. Awake at three a.m. worrying about problems? Too rajasic. During yoga class, are you giving up on a pose without trying? Tamasic. Striving hard because the person on the next mat does a pose well, even though it hurts your wrist? Rajasic. Gauging these tendencies helps you know when to back off and when to push harder.

The benefit of working toward the balanced sattvic state is improved mental and physical health. When in a sattvic state of mind, you'll find it easier to care about yourself and others, and to keep a calm, level-headed outlook in all circumstances.

KARMA: WHAT GOES AROUND COMES AROUND

At the gym people often say, "I missed yoga for three weeks and now I'm so stiff!" Or, "I stopped running and now I get out of breath so easily." This is a predictable cause and effect. Cause: You stop stretching. Effect: The body feels tight. Cause: You stop running. Effect: Your cardiovascular system declines.

Cause and effect also has a moral component, which Hindus call karma. This moral law of cause and effect means that your actions – good and bad – will sooner or later be appropriately rewarded by the universe. This may happen instantly or years later. Or, as Hindus believe, you might carry your karmic balance from one incarnation into the next.

Other religions hold similar beliefs. Christianity rewards your accumulated life choices with heaven or hell. Wiccans believe in the threefold law of return, which states that your actions come back to you three times over. Islamic law – cutting off the hand of a thief, for example – is an effort to formalize karma legally. Cause: You steal. Effect: Goodbye, hand. Most non-religious people also have a strong sense of right and wrong and the importance of justice. When people watch movies, they often revel in a villain's comeuppance, or an honorable underdog's pay off. These are examples of people reaping their karma.

Okay, lots of things happen that we don't think we sowed. A health-conscious person gets cancer. A cautious driver is paralyzed by a drunk driver. Hindus explain these unfair-seeming incidents with past life karma. Westerners, myself included, have a harder time with this idea.

So I don't try to figure out what's carried from one life to the next. Instead, I focus on the way karma plays out in easy-to-understand ways. If I'm unkind or dismissive to people, I'll soon have few friends. If I stop paying my mortgage, the bank will take my house. Cause. Effect. It's worth slowing down and taking action with the likely results in mind. Whether you're embarking on a new venture or about to say something less than kind to your spouse, pause and ask yourself, what will this action sow? What kind of karma will this action bring?

MANTRA: YOUR SPIRITUAL SECURITY BLANKET

My first experience with mantra – not counting reciting prayers for penance – was being initiated into transcendental meditation at the age of 16. The old purple Victorian house that had been converted into a meditation center intrigued me. I pondered the mysterious goings-on inside. So I saved up $125 for my initiation and even refrained from using mind-altering substances for the requisite two weeks, an unthinkably long time in that stage of my life. It was all worth it. During what seemed, at least to my teenage self, a mystical and elaborate ceremony, my teacher whispered a secret mantra in my ear.

Many years later, through the magic of Google, I learned that the secret mantras were based on age, gender and date, so that all the other 16 year-old girls got the same mantra that year. But no matter. I only rigorously followed TM for a short time, but the mantra has lasted me decades. I use it to help me focus. I silently repeat it during meditation. It's helped me stay still for medical procedures. My mantra figures into my life at least weekly, if not daily. So I highly recommend a mantra.

A mantra can be a sound, syllables or words repeated over and over. This technique is used by various spiritual traditions to focus the mind during meditation. Catholics say the rosary. Buddhists chant prayers. Some people use affirmations. Mantras can be repeated silently or aloud.

Some yoga studios host kirtans, which are events where people get together and sing mantras in a call and response style. These Sanskrit mantras generally glorify the various Hindu gods and goddesses. Few people in western yoga studios are Hindus, but many find inspiration in the positive attributes of the different gods. Or they enjoy singing in a group. Many find the simple, repetitious tunes calming.

You don't have to be initiated into anything to find a mantra of your own. Instead, you can pick one or more. It can be syllables or words, in your own language or another. While I've always kept my mantra secret, I will divulge that it is a couple of syllables with no meaning, as far as I know. I recommend that you keep your mantra secret, too. It's more personal and powerful that way. Sharing secrets dilutes them. And some people are all too willing to poke fun at secret mantras. Respect your mantra, keep it close to your heart, and it will serve you well.

KLESAS: KNOW YOUR AFFLICTIONS

In the Yoga Sutras, Patanjali identifies five klesas, or afflictions, which cause all sorrows and discontent. Unfortunately, they're qualities that most people have in abundance. Here are the five culprits: ignorance, attachment, aversion, pride or ego, and clinging to life. Ignorance is the umbrella over all the klesas, because if you were more spiritually knowledgeable, you wouldn't suffer the other four afflictions.

Attachments and aversions are likes and dislikes, from mild preferences to full-blown addiction. Who doesn't have likes and dislikes? Nobody I know. But some people get less upset than others when things don't go their way. That's the problem with likes and dislikes. You can be perfectly content as long as you get what you like and avoid what you dislike. But as soon as those two sets are reversed, you suffer. If you can work on being less invested in favorites and less hateful towards those people, places and things you like the least, you will feel more peaceful.

As far as ego, people identify with the titles and roles in their lives. Instead of being a soul who's temporarily experiencing a human body, you think you're a father, a banker, a yoga teacher, a friend. What happens if you lose your job? Your children? Your friends? Your health? Who are you then? You suffer when you lose the roles you identify with so closely.

Clinging to life, the last klesa, is the hardest for me to imagine overcoming. My immediate reaction is, of course I cling to life! What do I want to be, dead? But this clinging can lead to unhappiness when I make too many choices out of fear. Tonight I was driving home after teaching classes. It was 32 degrees, unusually cold for Portland. I drive a station wagon. People shivered at bus stops. It occurred to me that I could stop and offer them rides. But I immediately thought, that stranger could have a gun. Maybe he'll carjack me and steal my 22 year-old car. And even if I overcame my fear of offering a stranger a lift, chances are the stranger would have the same fear. He or she would worry about being abducted by a strange woman.

I'm not saying I should have stopped and coaxed strangers into my car. I'm just pointing out one small way that clinging to life provokes uncomfortable thoughts and feelings, even when my life is in no immediate danger. Multiply that little situation by 100 per day, and you get an idea of how subtly fear can permeate everyday situations.

So what can you do about the klesas? You can start with a gentle inquiry into your motives. You can pay more attention to how you make decisions. Are you deciding based on fear? Or on over-identification with your own self or roles in life? Are you letting your petty likes and dislikes get in the way of your happiness?

It's easy to feel defensive about letting go of preferences, or of the titles and accomplishments you worked so hard to get. But ultimately, everything changes. And clinging to your roles, preferences, youth, and, ultimately, your life, is futile and leads to sorrow.

SAVASANA: RELAX LIKE A CORPSE

At the end of most yoga classes, everybody lies down in savasana, or corpse pose. The idea is to make like a corpse, lying still and relaxed and not having any worries. While this seems like it would be the easiest pose, many people find it difficult. Of course, your breath, fidgety parts, life energy and busy, busy mind clearly divide you from a real corpse.

Some people claim that corpse pose is a boring waste of time. I've known a handful of yoga students who leave class right as corpse pose begins. They're busy people with better things to do than lie around in a yoga studio for five more minutes. If they try to do savasana, their minds race and escalate their anxiety.

Of course the busier you are, the more you need rest.

Some people almost never rest. Especially nowadays. Electronic devices foster other people's sense of entitlement to your constant availability. Can you ever relax alone, or with one companion, without responding to the demands of five or ten others? For some folks, spending five minutes on their back in yoga class might be the quietest thing to happen all week.

Ideally in savasana, you relax both your body and your mind. Thoughts may pass through, but you let them go without fixating on them. Yoga master BKS Iyengar recommends pausing after the exhalation if your mind is super busy.

Savasana is a time of integration. After spending an hour or so doing active asanas, savasana lets you integrate new physical and emotional feelings that came up during practice and new knowledge you might have learned about individual poses. It's also a time of energetic integration. Poses move energy through the body. Then you rest and let that energy settle and the blockages heal.

For me, savasana has yielded wonderful epiphanies and insights. Many times, an answer has come to me in corpse pose. I figure out how to solve a problem in my life. I've had fully formed visions of paintings and solutions to plot holes in my fiction writing. When I manage to let everything relax and settle, answers bubble up from my unconsciousness. If I'd instead remained busy, I don't know when or if these solutions would have managed to get my attention.

NADIS: ENERGY CHANNELS

You might have heard – or experienced firsthand – that doing yoga poses can free blocked energy in the body. But how does this energy move through you? According to yogic texts, the body has 72,000 energy channels. They're called nadis, which comes from the Sanskrit word "nad" for "flow" or "vibration."

People who have had acupuncture are familiar with the idea of invisible meridians running through the body, connecting their disparate parts. These are the same as nadis. Some are large and carry a lot of energy. Some are very small and obscure. I don't know if all 72,00 nadis are named. Most scholars seem to find only a handful especially important.

Of these, three reign supreme. The sushumna is the central nadi, which runs up the spine to the crown of our heads. When somebody says their kundalini has awakened, they mean that a great deal of latent spiritual power coiled at the base of their spine has suddenly come to life and is shooting from chakra to chakra up this central channel. This nadi is the autobahn to enlightenment.

The other two main nadis are the ida and pingala, the left and right energy channels, which are polar opposites. They spiral round and round the sushumna nadi, finally meeting up at the third eye. The ida/pingala opposition is very similar to the idea of yin and yang. Ida, which originates on the left side of the central nadi, is identified with coolness, the moon, mental processes, the color white and the feminine. Pingala, the righthand nadi, is active, warm, solar and male. One or the other of these two nadis is dominant at any given time. And most of us tend more toward one or the other throughout our lives.

If you want to determine which nadi is dominant, try alternate nostril breathing. Usually one side is doing most of the breathing. Regularly practicing alternate nostril breathing is also the best way to balance the main nadis.

Like chakras, obviously nadis don't show up on X-rays. But even if you don't believe they exist in a subtle energetic body, as stated in yoga texts, you can still benefit from contemplating the right and left nadis as a metaphor for the need to balance different aspects of your personality.

MUDRAS: YOGA FOR HANDS

Mudras are positions, usually of the hands, with symbolic meanings. Hindu and Buddhist statuary often portray the gods with their hands in mudras. Depending on how the Buddha is holding his hands, he might be expelling negativity, showing compassion or calling for witnesses to the truth.

You can use mudras to influence your mindset and mood. This at first sounds farfetched. How does the way we hold our hands affect how we feel? But just as crossing your arms and slumping feels different than standing tall and opening your chest, changing your hand position can alter your attitude.

The most common mudra used in yoga is anjali mudra, which is simply touching your palms together in front of your heart. This is also called prayer hands. In many cultures, this position denotes reverence and devotion. So does joining the hands together in front of the heart invoke these feelings because this mudra reminds us of prayer? Or did people start joining their hands to pray in the first place because this mudra invokes the feeling of reverence? I don't know, but for many people, it works.

The word "mudra" means "seal." According to yogic philosophy, joining the fingers creates a circuit which contains your prana, or life energy, rather than allowing it to dissipate. Depending on what you need at a given time, you can arrange your hands to boost and seal in that particular kind of energy. Hundreds of mudras exist, from very simple to complicated.

Gyan mudra is another common yoga hand position. In this one, you join the thumb and index finger and outstretch the other fingers. This mudra symbolizes the connection between the individual and the divine. When you're feeling all alone in the world, you can try intentionally joining the thumb and index finger and see if you feel more connected. It's also useful for boosting memory and mental clarity, and easing anxiety and depression. Statues often depict the Buddha with his hands in gyan mudra.

According to yoga teacher and psychologist Kelly McGonigal, mudras help embody the traits people aspire to. Instead of seeing yourself as lacking bravery or compassion, you can arrange your hands in the appropriate mudra and start to conjure up that trait within. McGonigal calls mudras "prayers translated into physical form."

MAYA: SEDUCED BY ILLUSION

I recently visited a church in a different neighborhood with a hardline Catholic priest. He warned the congregation about the distractions we must avoid: flesh, the world and sin. I found myself snickering in the pew. What on earth is left, I thought.

But this is essentially the a common view among religions. Maya, which is Sanskrit for "that which is not," is usually translated as "illusion." In Hinduism, the whole temporary, material plane is considered illusion. The atman, or soul, is what lasts. In Christianity, the body is temporary, the soul endures. Whether the religion professes one incarnation and then off to heaven or hell, or many incarnations and then liberation from the wheel of death and rebirth, the idea of temporal versus spiritual is basically the same.

Most people tend to identify with the temporary all or most of the time. And who can blame them? Meditating and praying are less likely to keep the lights on than working to earn money. With all the pressures of work, family, friends and taking care of each other, it can seem impractical to focus too much on the spiritual. And with all the temptations of good movies to see, delicious things to eat and drink, sex, gossip, advances in status, new clothes, artistic accomplishments and whatever else floats your boat, contemplating the spiritual aspects may seem like a drag.

But strangely, finding a connection with the spiritual is your best hope for security. Even though it's invisible and impossible to prove, faith is one of the strongest things we have going for us as people. Fortunes, homes and relationships come and go. Wars break out and displaced people lose everything they once took for granted. In times of real trouble, having a spiritual life suddenly becomes practical. It can help you retain some calm, hope and sanity.

Modern yogis live in the modern, usually urban, world. So you have to keep one foot in the temporary and one in the permanent. Even as you perform and enjoy your daily duties and pleasures, it behooves you to take a more panoramic view. Christians keep in mind that eventually they'll face their eternal reward (or punishment). Hindus try to avoid acquiring bad karma that will lead to lesser rebirths. If you're not religious, you can still think of the generations to come. Do your actions right now bode well for those people, animals and landscapes of the future?

One of my favorite cemetery markers is a bench in Portland's Lone Fir Cemetery that says, "This wasn't in my schedule book." In the context of a graveyard, the idea of a schedule book seems absurd. But how many people feel like they *are* their job titles and accomplishments? That they *are* their fashion choices, musical tastes, political leanings and a whole collection of other temporary, worldly attachments? Now is the time to cultivate that deeper view.

PRANA: LIFE ENERGY

Here's a great example of the western commercialism of yoga. Google "prana" and the main thing that comes up is a high-end yoga apparel company. But long before branding, prana was the name of the life energy that animates your body. While some eastern cultures have a word for prana – the Chinese call it "chi" or "ki" – there's no direct English translation.

In one way, prana seems abstract because you can't see it. But you can sure see its absence. If you've ever been with a person or animal as they die, you've seen this amazing change up close. One moment, there's the person or dog or cat you know and love. The next, they breathe their last exhalation and suddenly...they're gone. Their body still lies there, but what's missing? Prana.

Yoga poses unblock energy channels so the prana can flow better. This works best if you hold poses for a longer time and relax into them, rather than moving quickly from one to the next. You might feel a kind of release after spending a minute or two in a deep hip opener. That's the prana moving through.

But you use prana in many more ways than just in yoga poses. Whether a person is a devoted yoga practitioner, an occasional gym yogi or someone who's never heard of yoga, everybody depends on life energy.

So, if you acknowledge that prana is what separates you from a corpse, you realize it's pretty important to take care of it. When you run around from thing to thing, working too late, sleeping too little, worrying and feeling depleted, that's your prana you're running down.

How do you manage and increase your prana? According to Swami Venkatesananda, prana enters people through meditation, sleeping, water and food, in that order. This, he said, is because you face the least interference from your ego while meditating or sleeping. Conversely, you lose the most prana through talking and sex, and through strong emotion. Another interesting way of dissipating prana is when you do something you feel forced to do when you really want to do something else.

A lot of the advice for optimal prana comes down to general rules of good health and common sense. To manage your prana, you need sufficient rest and healthful and easily digested food. Manage your stress. Be careful about what you say and who you sleep with. Everybody's heard this a bazillion times before. But if you think of it in terms of respecting your precious life energy – the thing that separates you from a corpse – perhaps you will be a little more careful.

BHAKTI: DEVOTION

Bhakti yoga is about reaching enlightenment through devotion to the divine. The bhakti path appeals to emotional types with huge hearts.

This path comes out of South Indian poems from the 7th to 10th centuries. Poets wrote love poems to God as though writing to a lover. Other devotional practices included singing songs celebrating the deity, wearing emblems and making pilgrimages to the deity's special places. Sacrifices of animals or vegetables were also common. The idea was to so fully celebrate the god that one would be subsumed by the divine.

Bhakti goes over better in some places than others. In the US, one of the most visible examples of bhakti, especially during the 1970s, was the Hare Krishna movement. When devotees danced, chanted and played music, that was a display of bhakti. And just like many people find public displays of affection embarrassing, so many regarded these public displays of devotion.

Another funny thing about the bhakti movement in the west: The religion perhaps best known for a personal relationship with God is Christianity. But many western yogis reject the religion they grew up with to adopt bhakti for Hindu gods. I've seen this in many yoga studios and Hare Krishna temples, Americans singing their hearts out for Hindu gods, while these same folks would scoff at singing in a Christian church. What gives?

My theory is that lots of people have lingering resentments towards the religions of their youth. You may have been forced to go to church, taught lots of rigid rules and internalized stuff you wish you hadn't. The god presented to you may have seemed far from lovable and cuddly. You may find it easier to accept somebody else's religion, especially in this multicultural era when other people's ways are so celebrated. But people from other cultures may also wish to escape their roots.

Once I was talking to a group of young Indian people who lived in the San Francisco Bay Area. I told them I'd visited India and how highly I regarded Indian culture. There was silence as they stared at me like I was a moron. For them, coming to the west had helped them escape the strict parts of being raised in traditional Hindu households.

My point is, what people want to celebrate is probably present in each religion, just as each has restrictions and parts that make us uncomfortable. Bhakti practitioners seem to keep their concept of God pretty simple, as in God is love. Most people can feel good about this notion.

Whether you're devoted to Jesus, Shiva, another god or something more abstract, you can incorporate devotion into your life with or without public displays. Say a simple, silent grace before meals, acknowledging your good fortune to have something to eat. Count your blessings and say prayers of gratitude. Lots of studies have shown that practicing gratitude is one of the best ways to avoid depression. Bhakti yogis – who constantly acknowledge their good fortune – usually seem pretty darn happy.

YOGA AND HINDUISM

Few American gyms decorate with statues or posters of Hindu gods and goddesses. But if you venture further into the yoga world, perhaps visiting yoga studios, you will probably see images of Hindu gods. While you don't need to be Hindu to practice yoga, yoga does spring from Hinduism. Many yoga teachers and students become fond of Hindu god images and may develop favorites.

The Hindu gods freak out some westerners. Perhaps you have a strong religious tradition of your own. Christians may worry about a slippery slope that slides down to the worship of graven images. Atheists might be annoyed by a focus on the spiritual. Others will wonder why Hindu gods have so many arms. Many will be confused about what downward dog has to do with Hinduism.

Rest assured, you don't have to trespass against your own religion to do yoga. If you find yourself in a class where the teacher suddenly leads students in a chant to a Hindu god, that doesn't mean you have to join in. You can sit quietly and listen, or think your own prayers to your own god.

I've had a couple of Christian students hesitate to go on yoga retreats because they were afraid they'd get stuck in a situation of heavy-duty Hindu chanting. And I've read about people who are afraid that even taking a single yoga class will get them involved in Hinduism. It's certainly worth asking questions about any retreat beforehand to make sure it's a good fit for you. But the worries about being captured by Hindus are overstated. Aside from some outlier sects like the Hare Krishnas, Hinduism is not a proselytizing religion. The Hindus don't want you. Since Christianity is a highly proselytizing religion, many people might not even realize that some religions aren't trying to add to their numbers. Some Hindus are annoyed that asana has been adopted in the west, separated out from the more spiritual aspects of yoga, and that yoga in general has been separated from Hinduism. But this isn't because they want to convert you; they just want credit for giving something great to the world.

Okay. Even if you are 100 percent devoted to your own religion, you might still be open to hearing tales of the Hindu gods. Each god and goddess is known for his or her own attributes and personality. By meditating on the stories of their strengths and trials, you might see your own situation in a new way. So in the next readings, we're going to examine the gods and goddesses you're most likely to come across in the American yoga world. Note, there are many other Hindu gods, and many that are just as important in India, but we're concerning ourselves with the ones that have caught on in the U.S.

Note that Hindus believe that all the gods are manifestations of the same divine, formless energy. So the gods are not in competition with each other. They're all really part of the same divinity. But it's hard to worship the formless, so Hindus personalize their devotion by conceptualizing divine energy in one form or another.

SHIVA: LORD OF YOGA

Shiva, who is considered the god of yogis, is a complicated fellow. He's the part of the Hindu trinity that represents death, destruction and dissolution. However, that's not as grim as it may sound to westerners. In Hinduism, death is a prelude to rebirth.

Shiva takes many guises. Sometimes he is shown as a family man, posing in posters with his consort Parvati and their elephant-headed son Ganesha.

In his king-of-the-yogis form, Shiva is a master of meditation and austerity. He strolls peacefully through the cremation grounds. He meditates cross-legged, wearing only a tiger skin loin cloth. For yogis, Shiva brings the best kind of destruction: destroying the ego and false identification with the body, dissolving attachments and bad habits.

Shiva also takes the form of Nataraja, a wild dancer whose dance represents the destruction and creation of the universe. In yoga, the pose Natarajasana, or dancer pose, is based on this form of Shiva.

How do you recognize Shiva in Hindu artwork? He's portrayed with blue skin, at least on his face and throat, and has a prominent third eye. The cobra around his neck signifies his triumph over poison. Three horizontal white lines of vibhuti, or sacred ash, are drawn across his forehead. In India, you see some of his followers wearing these same lines. Shiva holds a trident and a two-sided drum, and rides a white bull named Nandi. Unlike other gods, Shiva is usually pictured in a simple natural setting, looking peaceful and wearing only an animal skin.

In India, the most devoted followers of Shiva are an austere bunch. They wear saffron clothes and smear their bodies with ashes. They meditate a lot. The path to Shiva is an introspective one.

Shiva has always been my favorite Hindu god, even before I started doing yoga. To me he represents keeping my cool in adverse circumstances. Many times I have pictured him serenely walking through the cremation grounds and tried to invoke just a little bit of that poise. He's the perfect mix of calm and awesome power. For anybody trying to master the fluctuations of the mind through yoga practice, Shiva's the supreme example.

GANESHA: ELEPHANT POWER

Ganesha is one of the most popular deities in both East and West. Apart from theological values, I think Americans like Ganesha because he's a happy, big-bellied elephant-headed god who enjoys sweets and pleasure. We can relate to him. If you're new to Hindu imagery, he's the first god you'll be able to recognize. Plus, for people in a Christian society, it might be easier to look at another culture's elephant-headed god than one with a human face. Worshiping an elephant just seems so out there, and not directly in competition with Jesus.

Ganesha, son of Shiva and Parvati, is a good-natured god of plenty. He's lord of success and wisdom and widely venerated as somebody who can remove obstacles in our lives. Almost all Hindus worship him, regardless of their sect. After all, who doesn't face obstacles?

The elephant-headed god is considered the lord of all existing beings. The story of how he beat his brother Kartikay to win this title demonstrates Ganesha's wisdom and humility. Whichever brother managed to race around the universe first would become lord of all existing beings. Kartikay got off to a fast start on his jaunt around the globe. Ganesha simply circled his parents, the mighty Shiva and Parvati.

In addition to the elephant head, Ganesha has several other noteworthy attributes. He's depicted holding a conch shell, lotus flower, an Indian sweet called a laddu and a hatchet to slash the bondage of desires. Sometimes he's shown with a trident or cobra, like his father, Shiva. He demonstrates humility by his choice of mount. Instead of riding a mighty bull like Shiva, Ganesha rides a mouse or rat.

HANUMAN: MONKEY GOD

Hanuman, better known to westerners as the Hindu monkey god, epitomizes devotion. Like many stories of gods, there are several versions. He might have been the son of the king and queen of the monkey gods. Or he might have been born to the god of the wind and Anjani, a celestial nymph cursed to appear as a monkey. Either way, despite Hanuman being a mischievous young monkey, he grew up to be a faithful servant to Lord Rama.

Hanuman plays a vital role in the Ramayana, a famous Hindu epic story. When the evil king Ravana absconded with Lord Rama's wife Sita, Rama sent Hanuman to do recon. Evil Ravana ruled the island of Lanka, now known as Sri Lanka. Hanuman, whose powers allow him to fly, flew to Lanka and located Sita. He then alerted Rama to her whereabouts. A huge and bloody battle ensued, resulting in Sita's rescue.

Rama's brother was horribly wounded in the battle. Hanuman flew off to the Himalayas to find the herb that could cure the wounded man. In addition to flying, Hanuman can also grow very large and strong. He didn't want to waste time locating the herb, so he picked up the entire mountain and flew back to Lanka, holding the mountain in one hand.

The yoga version of what westerners refer to as the splits is called Hanumanasana. It's named after when the monkey god stretched out his legs to leap from India to Lanka, which is about 16 miles at the closest point. The low lunge position that's halfway to the splits is named Anjaneyasana after Anjani, Hanuman's mom.

Hanuman embodies the idea both of selfless service and devotion. Hindus also revere him for his perseverance and physical strength. India is full of Hanuman temples, and Hindus often sing the hymn "Hanuman Chalisa" in times of difficulty.

My friend Jenny Gallagher told me one of her favorite Hanuman stories. The other gods thought Hanuman was too proud of his talents, so they removed his ability to remember them. But in dire situations, when he needed to fly or grow very large or small, his mother reminded him of his abilities. "I love how that helps me to remember to balance between humility and strength for the greater good," Jenny said.

Often Hanuman is pictured tearing open the skin of his chest to reveal the faces of Rama and Sita, meaning that they are in his heart. His devotion to them never falters. If you close your eyes and look inward, what do you see in your heart? To what are you unfalteringly devoted?

VISHNU: RELAXING ON A SERPENT SOFA

Within what can loosely be called the Hindu trinity, Vishnu is the peace-loving preserver of life. Usually he's pictured standing on a lotus flower or reclining on Adisesha, his giant serpent, while his consort Lakshmi massages his feet. It's a good life for a god.

However, when things get out of hand on earth, Vishnu incarnates to restore order. His earth births include a fish, a turtle, a boar, a dwarf, and a lion/man hybrid. His most famous incarnations are as Rama, Krishna and Buddha. Some people have also suggested that Jesus was an incarnation of Vishnu. The idea is very similar to that in Christianity: God is born as a man (or woman, turtle, boar, etcetera) and accomplishes an important mission on earth. Only in Hinduism, this has happened many times. Hindus still await Kalki, an incarnation of Vishnu which has yet to appear. He will apparently be seated on a white horse.

While some of Vishnu's incarnations are regularly seen in western yoga studios, Vishnu as Vishnu is not as popular. To identify him, look for these attributes: blue skin and four arms holding a conch shell, a discus, a lotus flower and a mace. He is sometimes pictured with his mount, Garuda, a giant eagle. Or on his serpent sofa, whose seven-headed cobra hood rises over Vishnu's head to protect him from the elements.

What can you learn from Vishnu? I think he embodies the idea of living a peaceful, content life while relaxing on his serpent couch. But at the same time, he's always ready to stand up and right wrongs when necessary rather than ignoring matters.

KRISHNA: THE MOST BEAUTIFUL GOD

Krishna, an avatar of the god Vishnu, is an extremely popular god in India and among western yogis. This blue-skinned god epitomizes joy, as evidenced by his pastimes of playing the flute and flirting with milkmaids.

The Hare Krishna movement that swept the US starting in the 1960s probably made Krishna the most famous, or infamous, Hindu god among Americans. His followers ceaselessly chant "Hare Krishna," which basically means Krishna is great. They do this as a show of bhakti, or devotion, putting Krishna above all else – including sex, food and sleep.

When I first met Hare Krishnas as a teenager, images of Krishna made a huge impression on me. I'd been raised in a church where every mass had me staring at Jesus crucified on a cross. This gory image traumatized me as a child. I was blown away to realize that Hindus conceived of a god who was happy, musical, and beloved by all. I'd never seen pictures of Jesus smiling and dancing. I suspect a lot of the young Americans who joined the Hare Krishnas were similarly impressed when they first encountered Krishna.

Hindus enjoy recounting Krishna's exploits as a child growing up in a family of cow herders. He was famous for his tricky behavior: stealing butter, hiding the clothes of bathing milkmaids and freeing cows at milking time. When he grew up, he battled demons with grace and style. One story has him defeating an evil multi-headed snake by dancing on its heads. He's most often depicted with his flute, and with Radha, Krishna's consort and the number one milkmaid.

The famous Hindu text Bhagavad Gita is 700 verses of Krishna and the young prince Arjuna talking philosophy and theology. Krishna spells out the path of devotion and selfless action. This scripture is an important guide for people living the life of bhakti who want to always keep their mind on the divine.

KALI: FIERCE MOTHER

The first time I saw an image of Kali, I was amazed by her ferocity. She's depicted with pure black skin, red eyes, her tongue sticking out and wearing a necklace of severed men's heads. I was immediately hooked. Growing up with the Virgin Mary as my female religious role model wasn't exactly empowering. Contemplating Kali's image was. Don't get me wrong. I appreciate Mary's gentle strength and serenity, especially as an adult. But sometimes a girl needs an example of the divine feminine who kicks ass.

Kali is a form of the divine mother. A fierce form. Think mother bear times one million. To her devotees, she's an extremely devoted mother.

Kali is the goddess of time and death. Her name comes from the Sanskrit word Kala, meaning time. Often she's depicted standing with her foot on Shiva's chest. The story goes that Shiva threw himself under Kali's foot to stop her from an extra-destructive killing spree. At which point she stuck her tongue out in astonishment to see Lord Shiva under her foot.

The goddess' other attributes include a sword in one of her four hands, a demon head in another, decapitated heads for earrings, a girdle fashioned from human hands and blood spatter on her face and breasts.

Two useful ways too meditate on Kali: When you're feeling lonely and unloved, imagine Kali's fierce motherly love directed at you. And when you're feeling powerless, downtrodden and like you're emanating the energy of a doormat, focus on Kali's image and invoke just a little of her ferocity.

DURGA: RIDING A TIGER

Durga is another fierce form of the mother goddess, though not as over the top violent as Kali. Durga was created to be a warrior.

The story goes that the demon Mahishasura repented for his misdoings so thoroughly that Shiva (or Brahma, in some stories) blessed him, making it impossible for a man or god to kill him. After this blessing, Mahishasura got too big for his britches and started raising havoc around the world. He had to be stopped, but it looked like Shiva had blown it by making the demon unkillable by gods or man.

So the gods Brahma, Vishnu and Shiva got together and created a woman who could defeat Mahishasura. Each of these gods, and many others, contributed their best weapons for Durga to wield in her ten arms. She also got a lion – or sometimes a tiger, depending on the story or image – to ride.

Mahishasura didn't believe he had anything to fear from a woman. In fact, when he saw her he thought they'd hook up. Instead, Durga and her big cat fought an epic battle against the demon and his army. It turned out that Mahishasura had shape shifting powers. So you might see images of Durga and her cat pouncing on a huge black buffalo, which is really the demon.

The name Durga means "invincible" or "inaccessible." Sometimes she is considered a fierce form of Shiva's consort Parvati. But when she goes onto the battlefield against the demon army, she is a single woman warrior, backed up by her lion alone. While both she and Kali are fierce goddesses, Kali seems more like a force of nature, beyond needing courage. Durga is more relatable, and is a useful goddess to think of when you feel like you're going alone into battle. She's not only brave, but she never doubts she will win.

LAKSHMI: GODDESS OF GOOD FORTUNE

The goddess Lakshmi brings fortune not only to people, but even to the other gods.

There's a story about the warrior god Indra offending Lakshmi with his arrogance. She got so disgusted with him that she left all the other gods and hid in the sea of milk. The gods started to have bad luck. People stopped worshiping them. Instead, the demons began to triumph.

And so the gods conspired to make Lakshmi return from the sea of milk. The best way, they decided, was to churn it up until she popped out. They tricked the demons into helping them. To churn the sea, they used a mountain as a pillar, placing it on the back of a giant turtle. The gods got on one side, the demons on the other, and they pulled Vasuki, the serpent king, back and forth around the mountain. It took them 1,000 years, but eventually treasures began to spring from the sea. These included amrita, or the sacred nectar, a magic wish-fulfilling cow, and Lakshmi, standing on a giant pink lotus flower and looking radiant.

Lakshmi took Vishnu as her consort. Luck returned.

The lesson here? Hard work is rewarded by good fortune. And when we are fortunate, we better not be arrogant about it or luck will desert us. Many Hindus believe that sincere worship of Lakshmi brings success, but that she withdraws her fortune from those who grow lazy.

Lakshmi is depicted in red or golden clothes. Often she stands upon a lotus, wears a lotus garland and holds a pot of gold coins. She may be pictured with her spiritual mount, an owl, or flanked by elephants or swans.

BANDHAS: ENERGY LOCKS

In your studies of yoga, sooner or later you'll hear about the bandhas. The word "bandha" is generally translated as "lock." These locks consist of physical and energetic contractions at certain parts of the body to direct the flow of energy. Some styles of yoga employ them more than others. Depending on the type of yoga, students may be directed to hold these locks throughout practice, just in certain poses and/or during breathing exercises.

The most basic is muladhara bandha, an energy lock around the genitals. This is very similar to doing a Kegel exercise, where you lift the pelvic floor and tighten the sphincter. It's often activated with the exhalation. Moving up to the abdominal area, the second most common bandha in yoga is uddiyana, which means flying upward energy lock. The feeling is of pulling the abdominals in and up. Jalandhara is the third most common bandha, which involves a constriction of the throat. This one is more likely to be used while sitting and doing breathing exercises, as it's awkward for postural alignment in most poses.

So what on earth are these energy locks for? Well, this is where it all gets pretty esoteric. Bandhas are supposed to help us redirect and manage our internal energy, rather than letting it all flow out and dissipate. Yoga teacher Jay Fields likes to think about how water in boating channels is moved through a system of locks. It's a way to move something powerful, like energy or water, against its natural flow. Activating mula bandha and uddiyana bandha in tandem keeps lots of energy contained in your midsection. Involve jalandhara bandha and the energy is contained between the genitals and the throat. People who like to work on energy healing of the chakras will find these locks useful. Some use the bandhas to activate their dormant spiritual possibilities.

Engaging muladhara and udiyana bandha can make certain difficult poses easier, especially those that involve balance and strength, like arm balance poses. If you ever played the slumber party game Stiff as a Board, Light as a Feather, you will understand. Certain types of muscular contractions seem to lighten the body for lift off.

You can get plenty out of yoga without knowing anything about bandhas. But if you want to take your practice deeper, experiment with this way to redirect and control your energy.

GURUS: LEADING US INTO LIGHT?

After writing a first draft of this piece about gurus, I read it to a friend who has more direct experience with gurus than I do. While I've had mentors and teachers, I've never given myself over to a person that I'd call a guru. My friend has. When she was younger, she was in a cult. She left it and regretted that alliance. Still, even after that interlude and its difficult psychological aftermath, she thought I was too hard on gurus. My friend still sees many positive aspects of the guru/devotee relationship.

Many people are confused by exactly what a guru is. One definition of the word holds that it's simply another name for a teacher. But others give more weight to the word. The syllables "gu" and "ru" are usually translated as dark and light, as in the spiritual light of the teacher dispels the darkness or ignorance in a student.

In many cases throughout history, guru relationships have worked beautifully. People have hugely benefited from wise teachers who were willing to help them develop spiritually and psychologically. If you're lucky enough to stumble upon an enlightened person who will help you this way, it could be the opportunity of a lifetime.

The problem is, how do you know if a given person can dispel your ignorance? Who is the real thing and who is a charlatan?

I recently attended a talk by Swami Chetanananda, who is a guru to many. In his personal experience, he said, gurus are essential. "But people in America are so allergic to the term guru," he said. He understands why this is the case. "The religion business has the lowest cost to produce of any business on earth," he said. "Bullshit is free. If they can sell it to you, it's 100 percent profit."

The guru problem reminds me of alcoholism. Just as most people taking their first drink don't expect to wind up in the gutter with only empty bottles for company, most people who go to a spiritual lecture don't expect to ever be prostrating themselves before the speaker, selling their house to keep him in Rolls Royces and cutting off contact with their nearest and dearest. Do you have the alcoholism gene? Do you have the blind devotion to a guru gene? You may not know until it's too late.

This all sounds pretty dramatic to people in yoga class. But unfortunately, guru sex scandals have rocked the yoga world in recent years. Several internationally famous, respected teachers have wound up accused of serious transgressions.

To be fair, the gurus are under a lot of pressure to spiritually guide their flocks. At the same time, the guru faces the temptations of a rock star—easy access to adoring groupies, who are ready to throw sex, money or anything else the guru's way in order to get closer. No wonder so many gurus end up embroiled in scandal.

Personally, I'm skeptical about how many truly enlightened folks walk amongst us. I don't think I've ever met any. However, I have met wise people with lots of insights to share who are still humans with the usual flaws.

You can also seek the guru within, whether you consider it the small voice of God, your purest self or your conscience. One group of yoga students – feeling burned by their teacher's sex scandal – produced a purple bracelet that says, "I am my own guru."

Another interesting guru question: Does the guru have to be alive? Some people consider Paramahansa Yogananda their guru, though he's been dead since 1952. Others treat Jesus as their guru, though he died about 2014 years ago. As Nitai Deranja, a Yogananda devotee, put it, "My guru has never been in his body since I've been active. In a way it's easier because we don't have personality to deal with."

ATMAN AND JIVA: TWO TYPES OF SOUL

Many westerners grow up with the idea that each person has an individual soul. Hindus also hold this belief, but with a twist. Hindus believe that atmans, or souls, temporarily inhabit a body. And then another body, and another. Distinct from your body and mind, the atman is the only part that lives on after the body dies. The atman is then reincarnated to a new body, just as a driver might outlast a car and get a new one.

As a teenager, I wandered into a Hare Krishnas festival in a local park. They'd hung up a big poster illustrating the atman's journey. The figures were arranged in a circle: a tiny baby turning into a boy, a young man, a middle-aged man, a senior, an elderly man, and then circling right back to the baby. The body changed and eventually died, but the soul cycled on. I remember this poster because it graphically depicted what's possible, and what some people believe.

So what is this soul? In Hinduism, the atman is made of the same stuff as the universal soul, or Brahman. So each person is a little piece of the divine going through their life and learning lessons before eventually learning enough to be freed from death and rebirth. At that time, the individual soul merges with the universal soul. Hindus regard souls as being more alike than Christians do. Christians tend to believe in ending up as individuated souls in heaven. Or, for real baddies, taking the eternal sauna.

Of course, when a soul is in a body, it becomes very attached to identifying with that body. Just look at how people bond over race, gender, and their perceived levels of attractiveness. Hindus call attached souls jiva, meaning "that which lives." Jivas believe in duality. That is, separateness from the divine. While the atman transcends space, time, name, form and causality, the jiva is bound by these five things.

Many people don't know what to believe. You may have been raised without religion, or with one you found unsatisfactory. Or your experiences may lead you to believe in the foolishness of all religions. Whatever you believe or don't believe, it's worth considering the viewpoint of the atman. What if instead of a corporeal human examining your spiritual side, you're really a soul temporarily having a human experience in a body? How would that change your priorities? Well, you'd probably want more sex and chocolate while you have the chance. But you might also view many of your concerns as petty and fleeting. You might feel more connection and compassion with all the people around you, who are also spirits trying to navigate the world in human bodies.

SAMSARA: CYCLE OF DEATH AND REBIRTH

Westerners are fond of saying, "You only live once." To a Hindu, this couldn't be farther from the truth. In Hinduism, the cycle of being born, dying, and reincarnated into a new body is called samsara. The chance for endless do-overs may sound appealing. But it's not a case of, "If I only knew then what I know now." The idea is you generally don't know. Your past lives are forgotten, except frustrating little pieces that may show up as déjà vu or in dreams. For Hindus, the point is to escape this seemingly endless cycle. Samsara has four major drawbacks: the recurrence of birth, disease, old age and death.

So how does evolution through reincarnation work? Remember the atman, or soul, that Hindus believe each person really is? When you die, your atman gets a new body. Who you become is based on a combination of your desires and your karma: what you want plus what you have earned. Maybe you want a Tesla, but your credit will only get you a '91 Camry wagon.

Past life karma is hard for many westerners to accept. It seems unfair and victim-blaming to say that somebody was born into poor and difficult circumstances due to his misdeeds in a former life. However, from the point of view of that person, being a Christian or Hindu could feel similar. Both have to work hard in this life to deserve either a good afterlife in heaven or a better birth next time around.

An atman can inhabit a surprising range of life forms, some with much more consciousness than others. The lowest form is aquatic life, followed by plants, reptiles and insects, birds, animals and humans at the top. Souls who behave as really great humans can come back as heavenly beings. Really bad ones can slip down the scale to sub-human levels. How many times are you reincarnated? The scriptures say countless times. Some Hindus believe that certain people reincarnate together, working out their karmic issues over multiple lifetimes.

MOKSHA: LIBERATION

So now that we've established that Hindus believe in an atman, or individual soul, which is reincarnated many, many times, you may wonder what is the end point of the soul's comings and goings? What happens when you escape samsara, the cycle of birth, death and reincarnation?

The final step after thousands – or according to some Sikhs, 8.4 million – of rebirths is moksha, or liberation from the cycle. And after 8.4 million times, life in a body could seem a little old. Hindus believe that when you finally completely neutralize your karma, your individual soul, the atman, unifies with the universal soul, or Brahman. Never to be born again.

The paradox of moksha is that you can't reach it until you give up all desires, even desire for liberation.

So what is the experience like? As far as I can gather, our individual souls are subsumed by the greater soul so that our independent consciousness ceases. While Hindus see this as deliverance, westerners sometimes see moksha as nihilism.

It's interesting to note the differences between how religions describe the afterlife. Male Muslim martyrs expect 72 virgins to await them. Mormons plan to remain eternally wedded to their spouses. Christians tend to picture harps and wings. While not all these images are equally exciting, they all promise some *thing*. Moksha is completely non-materialistic to the point where you don't even have our own soul anymore. It's such a different concept to wrap your head around that most westerners will never quite understand moksha's attraction.

DHARMA: DOING OUR DUTY

Hindus, Buddhists, Jains and Sikhs all use the term dharma or dharm, a word that has many interpretations. The Sanskrit word comes from a root which means to keep, hold, support or maintain. It's often used to describe natural or cosmic law, and is also used as a word for religion. Hindus consider it a mode of conduct which leads to spiritual advancement.

In India, the concept of dharma helps maintain the social order. People believe they have a place in – and a use to – society in accordance with natural law. This is very different from an American mindset where many people grow up believing they can pursue any career and, if they don't like it, start over once, twice or countless times. Historically, the idea of dharma made it much easier to justify India's caste system. It helps to keep peace in a very crowded country by focusing people's minds on behaviors that uphold the social order, such as religion, duty and vocation.

Americans – including me – chafe at the idea of staying in our own places to maintain order. However, the tradeoff is that more people seem to feel content. The problem with always striving for more is that there's a limited number of slots available for CEOs, movie stars, presidents, bestselling writers, astronauts and many of the other jobs most Americans feel best suited for. Which results in lots of unhappy clerks, bus drivers and baristas.

When I visited India, I was surprised by how seriously people took the idea of duty. I'd thank someone for doing me a service and he'd look at me kind of funny and say, "It's my duty." As though thanking him didn't make sense. They seemed to more fully embrace the nuances of their roles in life, rather than thinking they were too good for their jobs and so were determined not to do them very well. While I'm not saying that lack of career mobility is a good thing, the absence of bitching and moaning was refreshing.

Another dharma-related idea is that your dharma changes with age. Each stage of life has a different natural focus. Youth is about education. Then you get to chase pleasure and money for a while. Eventually, once your hormones have died down and your children are grown, you focus on your spiritual life and getting right with God.

Overall, I like to think that everybody has particular talents and a purpose in life, and that if you can pursue what you're doing with dedication, joy and service, you can be content. And social order is important, even though it can be confining. I mean, what would happen if you didn't feel like stopping at red lights so you accelerated? Some amount of conforming to rules makes it possible for humans to live in a group without harming each other more than we do.

SAMSKARA: THOSE DARN PATTERNS

The Sanskrit word "samskara" has a couple of meanings. One is a rite of passage, such as a wedding or baptism. But the definition we'll concern ourselves with here is samskara as thoughts, impressions and, especially, patterns.

Everybody has certain default things they do. These might be a type of relationship you repeatedly find yourself in, or a way of coping by drinking or overeating, or a habit of getting lazy in winter and sitting on the couch too much. Everybody also has at least a few good habits, such as kindness, generosity or commitment to beliefs. But where do these come from?

Hindus believe that as you experience something, the unconscious mind immediately forms an impression, or samskara. So each person has countless samskaras, some that are more powerful than others, due to frequency or intensity of the impressions. Many also contradict each other, as experiences with the same phenomena might have different results. This all sounds pretty reasonable to most westerners. Until we add in the part about samskaras being passed from life to life.

Hindus believe that babies are born with a whole set of samskaras, resulting in likes, dislikes, tendencies and habits that will soon reveal themselves. If you don't believe in reincarnation, you can think of this as nature and nurture. Some stuff you're born with, some stuff you acquire along the way.

Everybody has habits. The problem is that many people want to change certain habits, but change often seems impossible. From the viewpoint of Hinduism, these habits keep you tied to samsara, the cycle of death and rebirth. Only by burning through all our samskaras will we attain moksha, or liberation from being constantly reincarnated.

Whether you want to avoid being reincarnated or you simply want this life to be better, you might want to examine your habits and figure out how to change them.

Swami Sivananda said people have virtuous samskaras and evil samskaras. The way to root out the undesirable habits is to replace them with good ones. He likened a set of habits to a plank full of nails. If you have a bad nail, you should choose a better habit and, as Sivananda put it, "place it on the top of the bad one and give a hard tap with a hammer. In other words, you should make a healthy, useful suggestion. The new nail will be driven in perhaps a fraction of an inch while the old one will come out to the same extent."

This is a slow process, which takes determination and commitment. But you have the rest of your life, or lives, to practice.

SANKALPA: SETTING INTENTIONS

You might have taken a yoga class where the teacher suggested you set an intention. In Sanskrit, this intention is called a sankalpa. The idea is that during a moment when your mind is quiet, you plant a seed of something you want to grow. Unlike New Year's resolutions and goal setting, this is a gentle, subtle process.

Along with gentleness, word your intention positively. When setting goals, people often think negatively, which is only natural since you're thinking of how you want to change. But thoughts of how you've failed in the past can bring up self loathing. A sankalpa is a new beginning. Instead of saying, "I'm going to stop gorging myself on ice cream like a pig," choose something positive and more general, like, "I make healthy choices." Notice this is phrased in the present tense. As soon as you form your sankalpa, the new beginning has begun.

There are a couple of main ways to determine your sankalpa. One relies on thought. The other, intuition. You can think long and hard about your deepest desires, and how to form a sankalpa that will take you there. This might be the best way for some people.

I'm most familiar with sankalpas from yoga nidra, a practice where you lie in savasana while a teacher guides a meditation. My nidra teacher, Jennifer Siegel, tells us at the beginning that we will be setting a sankalpa, but not to decide yet what it is because we might pick the wrong one. So I try not to think about it, but of course I am turning over various intentions in my mind. Then a few minutes later, she suddenly instructs us to form a sankalpa. Sure enough, my mind has surprised me several times by coming up with something different than I had been planning. For example, one time I had decided on some ego-driven sankalpa like, "I excel at everything." But when she suddenly told us to set the sankalpa, I came up with, "I'm real." Some unconscious part of me had realized that a person who's set on excelling at everything – even during a passive, deep meditation – probably needs to get real and notice what's really going on rather than mowing down items on the to-do list.

If you want to try setting a sankalpa, wait for a quiet moment during relaxation or meditation and check in with what you really want. Make it short, phrased positively and in the present tense. It might also help to visualize your sankalpa as an image or a feeling. Check in on it later: a few hours later, the next day, the next. Does it still ring true? Can you feel its quiet power?

Your sankalpa may change. Maybe you attain your immediate intention. What's underneath? Sankalpas can deepen over time.

Why is it important to set an intention? Because you grow towards what you believe. As yoga teacher Rod Stryker puts it, the chief architect of life is the mind. Where you put your attention, your life will follow.

ABHYASA: PRACTICE!

The late yoga teacher Pattabhi Jois was often quoted as saying, "Practice and all is coming." His emphasis was firmly on abhyasa, a commitment to regular yoga practice. Just as you won't get very good at speaking French or playing the violin without practice, neither will your yoga improve without practice. And by "improve" I don't necessarily mean mastering difficult poses – though that might happen, too – but becoming more comfortable in your body and less ruled by constant and unruly thoughts and emotions.

Yoga students often return to class after a long hiatus. Maybe they got busy with their children or work or travel. Usually they say how much better they feel after doing yoga and are mystified or annoyed with themselves that they went so long without making time for their practice.

Why do people resist something that makes them feel better? Because much as you might love yoga, it's not always bliss. Sometimes you're busy or tired. Something hurts. You get bored of certain poses or they bring up uncomfortable feelings.

Consistency is important, so aim to make commitments you can keep. Can you realistically take a yoga class two or three times per week? If you're practicing at home, is it likely you'll stick to an hour every day? If not, how about half an hour? Ten minutes? Doing a short yoga practice with great consistency integrates it more firmly into your life than a weekly yoga marathon.

My friend yoga teacher Jay Fields gets impatient with people who say they are too busy to practice. "Really?" she asks in her book *Teaching People, Not Poses,* "What on my to do list is possibly more important than taking the time to anchor myself in my own presence?"

You don't need to worry how your practice turns out. Maybe it will be transformative and exhilarating. Maybe it will be boring or difficult. The more you choose to practice, regardless of the outcome, the more rooted your practice becomes in your life.

VAIRAGYA: NON-ATTACHMENT

Of equal importance to practice is vairagya, or non-attachment. This means committing to your yoga or spiritual practice but not getting hung up on the results. For example, don't say, "If I can't perfect my handstand by April I will give up yoga." Instead, keep practicing until April. When April comes, keep practicing.

You might have heard the saying "Let go and let God." It's kind of like that. Do your practice, let go of any expectations, see what happens.

Vairagya is the practice of letting go of things that lead you away from the spiritual. Namely, desires and aversions.

Non-attachment isn't easy. Desires and aversions attach you to people, places and things. The non-attachment process happens as you become aware of the things you are attached to and slowly start to loosen your hold. When you experience true non-attachment, you have sincerely lost your desire. It's different than, say, an ex-smoker having to talk herself into a dislike for cigarettes when secretly she wants to smoke a whole pack. With non-attachment, the connection to cigarettes is severed, so that the ex-smoker feels neutral. She neither desires them nor has a panicky aversion caused by the fear that she might start smoking again. In my own experience as an ex-smoker, I know that non-attachment can come and go. Most days I'm neutral and unafraid of picking up my old habit. But sometimes, many years after quitting, desire rears its head and yearningly sniffs for cigarette smoke. So much for doing things perfectly.

How do you work with desire and aversion while practicing yoga postures? My friend yoga teacher Kimberly Dark inspires me here. When she takes a yoga class, she figures her practice that day is to do what the teacher says, as far as she is able. She tries to check her opinions at the door. I try to remember this when taking classes. Instead of categorizing poses into ones I like and ones I dislike, I try to do each pose as it comes along. If one is difficult or I feel like I can't perform it well, I try to let go of any feelings of inadequacy and move on to the next one. It also helps to not look around too much at the other students. Comparing yourself – whether you think you're better at a pose or worse – just feeds desire and aversion. This is also true in most other areas of life. Non-attachment is a surer road to peace.

SATSANG: SPIRITUAL COMMUNITY

The Sanskrit term "satsang" means gathering together for the truth. It's used to refer to a spiritual community, sometimes led by a guru. The group may meditate together, ponder spiritual texts or do yoga.

So what is a spiritual community and what's the point of having one? Validation and moral support are two good reasons. Whatever's important to you is reinforced by the company of like-minded people. Only another stamp collector will understand why you spent four grand on that British penny black stamp. Other drug addicts understand how you traded your life for drugs. Other dachshund breeders will agree about the superiority over other breeds. And other yoga practitioners understand the point of spending an hour focusing on breathing and balancing your body's energy flow by arranging yourself in different shapes.

But when you mix up these groups, you might get the opposite of validation. Maybe the dog breeder thinks the stamp collector is wasting money. The stamp collector thinks the yogi is wasting time. The yogi thinks the drug addict is wasting life.

Take a look at your life. Do the people around you share your spiritual path? Or at least give you moral and emotional support for the path you've chosen? Whether your path involves yoga, church, a 12-step group, hiking in nature or any of the myriad other ways you might view spirituality, your spiritual part thrives through acceptance and sharing. The opposite is also true: if you hang out with people who mock or belittle your beliefs, your flame of faith can flicker.

I'm not suggesting only being friends with people just like you. But it's a huge help to have at least a handful of people who relate to your spiritual beliefs. And even if you do yoga for stretching rather than spiritual reasons, associating with other yogis is beneficial. In general, people who practice yoga are interested in at least trying to live happier and healthier lives. You'll find fellowship and encouragement for your efforts to be calmer and more balanced. And that's a big step up if you're usually surrounded by people who settle for indifference or misery.

FRIENDLINESS

A few years ago, a couple of women showed up in my class at the gym. These two friends were refugees from a yoga studio in town that required a solemn demeanor. For them, a yoga class was a fun time when they met at the studio, chatted for a few minutes before class started, then enjoyed doing poses together. But the studio had a different idea: absolute silence. They were repeatedly reprimanded for speaking to each other.

I can see the benefits of both approaches. The studio provided an oasis from a busy world, a chance for inner contemplation free of noise pollution. Many people crave this quiet journey inward.

But my classes aren't like that. Students talk back. Sometimes they groan about a pose, or occasionally make comments unrelated to yoga. We enjoy some quiet time in class, but we also interact. And anyway, who would I be fooling if I pretended we were at some kind of sanctified retreat? We're gym yogis. During class we routinely hear weightlifters drop dumbbells (Who raised these people?), slam medicine balls on the floor, hawk up the contents of their lungs and slap their feet on the treadmill. The whole class has dissolved into giggles during savasana due to one weightlifter grunting as though straining toward orgasm.

Occasionally I worry that I'm not reverent, solemn and quiet enough to be a yoga teacher. So I take heart in my favorite yoga sutra, which describes how to behave toward other people.

Here it is: "By cultivating attitudes of friendliness towards the happy, compassion for the unhappy, delight in the virtuous, and disregard toward the wicked, the mind stuff retains its undisturbed calmness."

I've definitely had times in my life where I've felt envious of the happy, thought the virtuous were annoying goody two-shoes, wanted to give unhappy people a wide berth and was either attracted to or judgmental of the wicked. None of which leads to a calm mind. Instead, I'm much happier and more tranquil when I cultivate good feelings for the happy, unhappy and virtuous, and neutrality toward the wicked. Coveting, contempt and judging are the fast track to an unhappy, isolated me.

I love this sutra because it prescribes friendliness and delight in other people's company. I want to feel this in my life, and I want my students to feel it in class. We are not separate little islands who have to exist alone and wounded. And if the yogis are right, our individual souls will all eventually merge anyway. So we might as well start loving and befriending each other now, in and out of yoga class.

ABOUT THE AUTHOR

Teresa Bergen is a yoga, group fitness teacher and personal trainer in Portland, Oregon. She writes about health, fitness and travel. Teresa has studied with many yoga teachers – some famous, some obscure – and they all taught her something. Her work appears in many online and print periodicals and she's the author of *Vegetarian Asia Travel Guide*. Find out more at www.teresabergen.com. You can write to Teresa at teresa.bergen@gmail.com.

www.ingramcontent.com/pod-product-compliance
Lightning Source LLC
Chambersburg PA
CBHW070300290526
45791CB00003B/1021